How to Break Bad News
A Guide for Health Care Professionals

How to Break Bad News
A Guide for
Health Care Professionals

ROBERT BUCKMAN, M.D.

with contributions by
Yvonne Kason, M.D.

The Johns Hopkins University Press
Baltimore

The Johns Hopkins University Press
2715 North Charles Street
Baltimore, Maryland 21218-4363
www.press.jhu.edu

Library of Congress Cataloguing-in-Publication Data

Buckman, Robert.
  How to break bad news : a guide for health care professionals /
Robert Buckman : with contributions by Yvonne Kason.
      p.   cm.
  Includes bibliographical references and index.
  ISBN 0-8018-4490-8 (h). – ISBN 0-8018-4491-6 (p)
  1. Physician and patient.   2. Interpersonal communication.
I. Kason, Yvonne.   II. Title.
  [DNLM:1. Communication.   2. Interviews–methods.   3. Physician–
Patient Relations.   W 62 B925h]
R727.3B83 1992
610.69′6–dc20
DNLM/DLC
for Library of Congress   92-10298

A catalog record for this book is available from the British Library.

This book is dedicated to

Dr. Alon Dembo:
a great doctor, a great man

and

Edward Joseph Kason:
inspiration, lovingly remembered

Contents

Acknowledgments

The influences of a large number of people (clinicians, researchers, and authors) have contributed to the evolution of the ideas in this book. In putting it together, I have collaborated closely on every topic with Dr. Yvonne Kason, whose Interviewing Skills course at the University of Toronto gave the Breaking Bad News course its first permanent home.

The Breaking Bad News course was originally based on ideas tested and developed into video scenarios with Dr. Peter Maguire of the University of Manchester, without whose gentle expertise I might have given up before I had really started. I learned most of my practical skills from my many mentors, particularly Dr. Eve Wiltshaw, Dr. Robin Skynner, and Jane Dorsett. There have been several beacons of perceptive intelligence (by which I mean that their opinions accord with mine) in particular: in clinical practice Dr. Eric Cassell, and in research Dr. Douglas Maynard – both of whom were also kind enough to review this manuscript and offer useful and constructive comments. Additional valuable input came from Dr. Brian Doan. Where a paper or book touches on several relevant topics, rather than repeat the reference several times, I have highlighted the work under "Further Reading" at the end of the chapter concerned.

I owe many other debts: to the many patients and relatives who taught me while they thought I was teaching them; to the unflappable Ian Montagnes at the University of Toronto Press; to

Peggy Kee, who kept me supplied with reprints, references, and literature searches even when I had no idea what I wanted; to the inventors of the Sharp notebook computer that allowed me to write anywhere anytime, thereby depriving me of any excuse for not writing; and finally to Anne Gardner of Microsoft for help in the desperate eleventh hour, without whom – literally – all would have been lost.

Videos: The teaching videos on which the Breaking Bad News course is based are published in Canada and the United States by Telegenic Videos, 20 Holly Street #300, Toronto, Ontario, Canada M4S 3B1, and in Britain by Linkward Productions, Shepperton Studio Centre, Studios Road, Shepperton, Middlesex, TW17 0QD, England.

Robert Buckman
Toronto 1991

How to Break Bad News

1 Introduction

Why this book is necessary

Case History: The following incident is a rare one in that it illustrates almost all of the most serious errors in breaking bad news in a single interview. It occurred on the North American continent in the late 1970s, and it would be comforting (but overoptimistic) to think that it could not happen today. The patient was Mark L., a factory worker, born in Europe and now in his late fifties, who was admitted for prostatic biopsy. He was in a two-bed unit on the ward. The senior surgeon came in and stood near the door, speaking to Mark and the patient in the next bed together. He first told the man in the next bed that he could go home, and that his biopsy showed benign hypertrophy. He then turned to Mark and said, without moving from his position at the door, *I'm glad to say you can also go home, but there's bad news as well – the biopsy showed cancer of the prostate.* The physician then left without further discussion. Mark later said that compared to all the difficulties he had to face subsequently (surgery, radiotherapy, and chemotherapy) nothing affected him as badly as that encounter and nothing left him so distraught and with so little idea of how to cope.

As health care professionals we all know that breaking bad news is a difficult and unusual part of our job. We also know that it is virtually inescapable and that there will be very few of us who do not, at some time, have to break bad news to a patient or relative, or offer support subsequently to someone who has just received it. Yet although the task is so common, there seem to be very few objective facts known about it or about how it should be done. Worse still, there is a forbidding taint to the subject. It is almost as if the idea of improving our ability to break bad news was taboo and not to be discussed in polite society. Teaching techniques of breaking bad news is almost as awkward now as teaching contraceptive practices must have been in the Victorian era. We all know that errors are common and misunderstandings frequent, but our society complies with the assumption (or rather the pretense) that we are all doing the job well.

In fact, most of us in clinical practice have not been taught very much (if anything) about the technique of breaking bad news. Furthermore, the psychologists and social scientists who carry out research in the subject and have the most data do not have to perform this task in daily practice. As a result, breaking bad news is something of an orphan. All professionals know that it is part of their responsibility, and yet it does not seem to belong to one discipline more than any other. There have been no previous textbooks written on the subject and there are no generally accepted guidelines on how it should be done most effectively. This book is our attempt to fill those gaps.

In the writing of this book, we are each drawing on our own experience in practice and in teaching gained over the last few years. Individually and together we have both been teaching communication skills to medical students for seven years, and together we set up and now teach a course in breaking bad news at the University of Toronto. It was partly at the urging of our students, who wanted a practical and comprehensible text on the subject, that we began writing this book (although we have designed it to be read by health care professionals in all disciplines and at all levels).

Our own experiences in practice – in medical oncology and in family medicine – have stimulated us to draw up guidelines that are, above all, practical. All the recommendations and hints in this book can be used (and are used daily) in busy clinical practice. As may be expected, perhaps, many of the examples in this book concern the diagnosis of cancer. This is not to imply that other diseases have a lesser impact on patients and family, but the selection reflects not merely our own case-loads but also the particular dread that most people experience when the word (or suspicion of) "cancer" is discussed. Obviously, the guidelines that we put forward are as applicable to other situations involving bad news as they are to the cancer patient.

In setting out the six-point protocol that is central to this book, we are not implying that this approach is the only one or even that it is unarguably the best. There are insufficient research data on the subject to define the best method of breaking bad news beyond dispute, and it is difficult to design or even imagine research studies that would settle the issue definitively. (However, it is reassuring to note that contemporary existing research does support an approach that is very similar to the one presented here.[1]) We are presenting these guidelines as an approach that is (1) practical and useful in daily clinical situations, (2) based on some consistent and coherent principles, (3) intelligible, (4) teachable, and, most important, (5) learnable. In other words, the protocol that we are describing is an everyday hands-on approach that can be described easily and can be passed on to juniors and trainees. In our view, that is at least a start, and is preferable to the present method (or lack of it), which consists mostly of random apprenticeship and serendipity and is the manner in which most of us in current practice learned whatever craft we now possess.

Despite that disclaimer and despite the dearth of objective research data, there is no doubt that breaking bad news is important, and becoming more important. A few decades ago, bedside diagnostic skills were the essential techniques of the real physician. Therapeutic interventions and doctor-patient dialogue were far less significant. Currently, although we cannot do without those bedside clinical skills, our ability to make a diagnosis also requires a full and detailed knowledge of ancillary tests, and our ability to treat requires a detailed and current knowledge of contemporary research. This body of knowledge increases the amount of information over which we must exert some mastery, and this, coupled with the rise in patients' rights to information and choice, means that all of us will be required to spend increasing amounts of time explaining aspects of clinical medicine to patients. If the news is bad and the implications are serious, most patients will wish for more information and more discussion than they will if the situation is straightforward and curable. These interviews, concerning bad news and its implications, are the ones that are most difficult for the health care professional, and it is for these situations that clear strategies and excellent communication skills are most crucial. It is our hope, as authors, that this book will enhance both.

Who should read this book?

This book is intended for all health care professionals – doctors, nurses, social workers, psychologists, counselors, chaplains, volunteers, or members of any other discipline – as well as for trainees and students. However, some of the material will be of greatest value to physicians, because in most areas of contemporary medicine the breaking of bad news is regarded as primarily the responsibility of the physician. This may or may not be a good thing, but it does seem to be the way the world works at present. Therefore, while most of the book may be interesting to all professionals, the protocol set out in chapter 4 is intended primarily for doctors (and medical students). That does not mean that it should not be read by others. In fact, understanding the protocol will greatly enhance the value of the support that can be given to the patient (or even the physician) later on by other professionals.

A brief note about the format

Ground Rules: Many of the practical tips in this book are reiterated as "Ground Rules." The whole objective of a ground rule is to offer a possible direction or option when there seem to be no immediate clues as to what to do next. Like all ground rules, they are neither absolute nor inviolable, but offer a potential track when the wilderness seems impassable.

Practice Points emphasize finer details. They are intended to illustrate options in the more complex dilemmas in which we all find ourselves involved from time to time.

Case Histories: all case histories are based on real patients, but of course all the names have been changed.

"Professional" and **"patient":** We use the word "professional" as an abbreviation for "health care professional," by which we mean members of any health care discipline (doctors, nurses, counselors, social workers, psychologists, chaplains, students, and all others). It is, in itself, a rather unattractive word, but it is a useful shorthand to indicate whom we are talking about. Similarly, we use the word "patient" to mean "the person with the illness." We also use "her or his" and "his or her" despite the clumsiness of the phrasing because there is no sexless pronoun for human beings.

Objectives

This book has three main objectives:

TO INCREASE THE READER'S RIGHT/WRONG RATIO

An expert in breaking bad news is not someone who gets it right every time – she or he is merely someone who gets it wrong less often, and who is less flustered when things do not go smoothly. This book cannot provide an infallible formula for getting it right (there is no such thing), but it may improve your success rate. In general, the most common problems are caused by relatively simple errors – faults in common courtesy, failures in listening or in acknowledging the patient's needs. This book, therefore, will provide you with various means of avoiding these common errors and of increasing your "right/wrong ratio." It will encourage you to look at the way you perform certain tasks (patterns of behavior that are often ignored in daily practice) and to see the consequences of those actions and the different options available. Whether each of us realizes it or not, as professionals we are constantly transmitting messages to our patients. We all need to be aware of what those messages are, and of the effect that they have, in order to reduce the incidence of unwanted side effects.

TO INCREASE YOUR COMFORT AND ABILITY TO SUPPORT

The professional's level of comfort in doing her or his job is an essential part of the equipment and expertise required for the task. It is not an item of personal luxury. If you are uncomfortable in doing a particular part of your job, you will have a tendency to back away from that situation, and this will be perceived by the patient as abandonment. Conversely, the more competent you feel, the closer you will be able to get to the patient. This is the first and most crucial element in supporting the patient. Thus, your own comfort is actually an integral part of your ability to provide good patient care. Increased confidence translates into increased competence.

TO ENHANCE LEARNING

Much of the most valuable education in breaking bad news comes, not from didactic teaching or even from good role models, but from patients and their relatives. Their feedback (whether it is praise, criticism, or gratitude) educates us all and helps us to distinguish adaptive and supportive responses to bad news from unhelpful ones (both the patients' and ours). Therefore, one of the major objectives of this book is to increase the reader's sensitivity to feedback – to encourage the reader to develop into a person capable of self-enhancement and of progressively increasing her or his own abilities and expertise, rather than an automaton who turns out "textbook" responses to any given situation.

Why this task is worth doing well

There are several compelling reasons for attempting to improve the standard of breaking bad news. First, it is part of the health care team's (particularly the physician's) job. Breaking bad news is not an optional add-on to a professional's specialist abilities; it is a mandatory part of his or her basic skills. The public expects it and is vociferous when it is not done well. The media constantly report complaints by relatives about the way patients or family have received bad news, often detailing the manner in which the doctor (usually) performed the job (*he seemed so cold* or *he was so insensitive ... almost brutal*). Of course, some of that dissatisfaction may be attributable to the news itself ("shooting the messenger"), but often the doctor's behavior may well have seemed cold and insensitive. In the great majority of cases, those doctors were not cold or insensitive (most doctors aren't) but they were uncomfortable, edgy, and embarrassed. They may well have been aware that they did not know how to carry out the interview effectively and supportively, and so may have backed off, attempting to end the interview quickly to reduce their own discomfort and sense of clumsiness. They may well have overused medical jargon in order to give an air of efficiency and professionalism to the proceedings, and thus may have added to the perception that they were impersonal or indifferent. In today's social climate, breaking bad news is a highly visible part of the professional's public profile.

Second, the law demands that this job be done well (with various levels of rigor depending on which country you practice in). The frequency of litigation varies from country to country, but there are two common factors in all parts of the world: (1) litigation is becoming more, not less, frequent and (2) the most common cause of litigation is failure of communication rather than true medical negligence. Of course, the avoidance of trouble is not the main reason for wanting to do the job well, but it is a powerful and practical secondary incentive.

Third, doing this task well enhances your own satisfaction in your professional life. Without it, looking after patients who are not recovering or who are incurable is tiring and may cause you

to suffer "burn-out" later in your career. If you can continue to
function well even when you are dealing with bad news, you will
last longer.

Individually and together these are compelling reasons for in-
vesting time and effort in improving this part of the professional's
job.

Should we tell the truth?

Having established, then, the idea that breaking bad news is an
important part of the job of all health care professionals, we now
have to consider a difficult ethical question: namely, when breaking bad news to a patient, are we under any obligation to tell the
truth? This issue has not always been a simple matter to decide.
Until recently, perhaps even a few decades ago, it was not regarded
as standard medical practice to tell patients the truth. Certainly
there have always been advocates of truth-telling – one early example was the French physician Samuel de Sorbière.[2] He suggested in 1672 that more truth-telling might be a good idea, but
thought that it might seriously jeopardize medical practice and
concluded that the idea would not catch on. For the following
four centuries, it seemed that de Sorbière was right. Ambivalence
about the principle of truth-telling was consistently shown in the
physician's absolute control over the amount of information transmitted to patient or family. In the 1950s and the 1960s, approximately 90 percent of physicians indicated that when the diagnosis
was cancer, they preferred not to inform the patients,[3] and there
were even published methods for evasion or overt deceit.[4]

This attitude was based on the widely held view that truth may
be damaging – that disclosure of the true medical facts may destroy
a patient's hope or motivation – and on an underestimate of the
number of patients who want disclosure[5] (one aspect that is still
a problem[6]). In fact, there is little convincing evidence that truth-
telling or awareness of a grave situation does serious harm,[7] such
as inducing despair or suicide.[8] Furthermore, despite physicians'
estimates, there has always been a high proportion of patients

who want to know the truth. The percentage varies from 50 percent to 97 percent, depending on the studies,[9] but independent of the nature of the disease[10] (for extensive surveys of the literature see McIntosh[11] and Northouse[12]). Furthermore, this preference holds despite any initial shock felt by patients on having their suspicions confirmed.

Patients, therefore, have been overwhelmingly and consistently in favor of hearing the truth, but until recently physicians were not in favor of disclosing it, and greatly underestimated the number of patients who wanted it. However, there has been a marked change in physicians' policies and attitudes over the last two or three decades. A repeat study of physicians in 1979[13] showed that practices had changed considerably since 1951. Whereas 90 percent of the physicians in 1951 did not disclose the truth to cancer patients, by 1971 90 percent did (as a general policy) and only 13 percent generally withheld truth (for a lengthier analysis see Billings[14] and Maynard[15]). Physicians have thus changed their attitudes in response to social pressures.

It is now generally held that all mentally competent patients have absolute rights (ethical, moral, and legal) to any medical information that they require or request. These rights come from three interrelated sources: the expectations of society in general, the recognition of truth-telling as part of the code of ethics of the medical profession, and case precedence in law. At present in this country, therefore, there is little or no controversy about the existence of the patient's right, although there are often difficulties deciding whether a particular person, in her or his individual circumstances, wishes to abrogate those rights.

However, the patient's rights do not solve all the problems of breaking bad news. The debate has now moved on from *"whether to tell"* to *"how to tell"*[16] or, more important, "how to share the information" (stressing the fact that this process is part of a dialogue, a two-way conversation, between the physician and patient, not a one-way pronouncement from physician to patient). Some clinicians feel that respect for the patient's right to know may have been embraced with excessive enthusiasm and that appropriate sensitivity to the patient's feelings may have been abandoned. It may be that unthinking and insensitive truth-telling is as delete-

rious, in its own way, as unthinking and insensitive truth-con-
cealment. Perhaps the best analogy comes from Simpson, who
suggested that truth is like a drug, and that it has its own phar-
macology.[17] Insufficient doses are ineffective and may harm the
patient's trust in the therapist; overenthusiastic scheduling may
cause symptoms of overdosage; and there are known cases of
idiosyncratic reactions, tachyphylaxis, and tolerance, as well as
occasional individuals who appear to be resistant to it. Thus, the
manner in which truth is shared may be an even more significant
predictor of the outcome than the simple fact that truth has been
told.

Clearly, whatever the proportion of patients who do want full
disclosure, as health care professionals we have to devise a method
of determining the individual's wishes and of tailoring our information-sharing to that person. This is the principle underlying the
protocol for breaking bad news set out in chapter 4 of this book.

Who should break the bad news?

The subject of whose responsibility it is to break bad news is also
a complex one. In theory, it is, like all aspects of a patient's care,
the ultimate responsibility of the senior physician (the consultant
or the staff physician) in charge of the patient. However, because
it is often an awkward task, because there are no established standards of practice, and also because of the logistic realities of on-
call schedules, it is quite frequently delegated to junior doctors, or
nurses. (In Britain in the 1970s, for example, most hospitals had
a policy that when a patient died, it was the senior nurse's job to
inform the relatives. Physicians and students were told that this
was not part of their duties, and did not even have the opportunity
to see how the nurses held these conversations.)

In our teaching experience in Toronto, we have heard many
examples from junior doctors and medical students which suggest
that delegation of the task often creates difficulties later on. Some
of those difficulties can be dramatic:

Case History: A woman in her early fifties died unexpectedly of a post-infarct dysrhythmia late at night. A fourth-year medical student was instructed by the resident to telephone the husband and inform him of the death. The student had joined the clinical unit that day and had not yet met with the husband, who lived a considerable distance from the hospital. The student made the phone call and the husband reacted aggressively, shouting and crying and finally cutting the call off abruptly. The student reported this to the resident, who then telephoned the husband several times over the next two hours. There was no reply. Fearing that the husband might have killed himself, the resident then called the local police, who broke into the husband's house, only to find that he had gone to stay with his brother.

Bad news (be it communicated to a patient or a relative) is material that must be handled carefully and with due precautions and skill. Examples such as the above suggest that the task should (ideally) be carried out by someone with expertise and experience.

Furthermore, the person who breaks the news should have some measure of continuing responsibility and commitment to the patient or relative. Breaking bad news is usually more than a "one-shot" event and there are often consequences and questions that will require further discussion. It is better for the patient if the person who breaks the bad news is the person who will be able to address at least some of these issues later. (As one perceptive surgeon put it: *I would no more ask my resident to do this than ask him to do an aortic graft.*)

In an ideal world, therefore, professionals would acquire expertise in conducting bad-news interviews from specific teaching early in their training, and would acquire experience from seeing good examples of these interviews before they have to hold one on their own. In practice, this does not happen (although with the development of specific teaching courses, it is becoming more common), and there are still many stories such as the one above. In our view, as teachers of this subject, a situation such as the one cited is unfair for both the giver and the recipient of the news and is likely to leave a major scar in the memory of both parties. Effective and supportive interviews about bad news are important enough to be the responsibility of a senior person who has the necessary skill and experience. It is hoped that this book will assist the professional to utilize her or his own experience to enhance the skills needed for this job.

SUMMARY

1   Breaking bad news is an important part of the health care professional's job and requires experience and expertise.

2   We have ethical and legal obligations to tell patients the truth – but the manner of doing so is an important predictor of the outcome of the interview.

3   Breaking bad news is a skill that can be learned and can be used in a busy clinical practice.

FURTHER READING

Maynard D. Bearing bad news in clinical settings. In: Dervin B, ed. Progress in communication sciences. Norwood: Ablex, 1991

2 Why Breaking Bad News Is Difficult

A definition of bad news

We all understand what bad news means, but often have great difficulty defining it. One definition that is useful in practical terms defines bad news as any news that drastically and negatively alters the patient's view of her or his future.[18] This definition implies that the "badness" of any bad news depends on what the patient already knows or suspects about the future. In other words, the impact of bad news depends on the size of the gap between the patient's expectations (including his or her ambitions and plans) and the medical reality of the situation. As we shall see, this definition also means that the impact of bad news cannot be judged until you know what the patient already knows and expects. This aspect will be examined further in the following parts of this chapter, showing how this view of bad news offers a useful technique for starting the interview.

Why bad news is bad

Naturally, most people do not want to be told that they are ill, and resent or even hate the prospect of their life-style and its opportunities being reduced or threatened by their state of health.

Equally, every physician (except the rare one with impenetrably thick skin) dislikes having to break bad news. We all know that it is difficult, and most of us also feel that to some degree we are incompetent or inept at it. (One highly experienced physician expressed the feelings of anxiety that never become completely resolved this way: "After thirty years as medical director of a palliative care unit, I still feel relieved when a patient says 'It's all right, doctor, I knew it was cancer anyway.' ")

However, it is most important to realize that much of that feeling of ineptitude and awkwardness is preset – it exists before the interview with the patient begins. Some of it is caused by the way our society currently views illnesses, some is the result of the patient's discomfort and of our consequent empathic experience of their pain, and some caused by our own professional training. It is worth reviewing these main sources of the professional's discomfort, since this may then enable the reader to see them as features of contemporary society and to take them less personally.

SOCIAL FACTORS

At the moment, most Western societies are going through a phase in which the greatest value and admiration is set aside for youth, health, and wealth. This is neither a good thing nor a bad thing (life may not necessarily have been better – or fairer – in societies where age was the most valued and revered human attribute); it is merely the way the world is in most of the developed nations. However, there is a price to be paid for this outlook, and that price is paid by those who do not have youth, health, or wealth – the elderly, the sick, and the poor. These groups are, to use a current word, "marginalized," meaning that they are perceived as outside the mainstream of society, on its fringes. Hence when we, as professionals, have to tell someone that they are ill, to some extent we are telling them that their stock of health is diminishing, that they are closer to being a member of a marginalized group, and that – through no fault of yours or theirs – their social value is being diminished.

Even when the illness is purely random (as many are) there is still a social taint to bad luck: people do not like to be contaminated by bad luck and are apt to be uncomfortable and resentful when they are told that it is happening to them. Thus, since our society values the sick less than the healthy, discussions about ill health implicitly carry overtones of social demotion. That demotion and the separation from the mainstream of everyday life are even more acute and painful when the bad news also carries the threat of dying. Even though the threat of dying may be a component of only a small proportion of interviews about bad news (depending on your specialty), it is worthwhile looking at some reasons why our society puts such a high price on the process of dying. This attitude to dying, in a covert way, colors society's attitude to all illnesses and disabilities, a matter we shall deal with later in this chapter.

PATIENT FACTORS

There are literally thousands of features of illness that patients may fear, and every human being has a unique and individual combination of fears and concerns. This topic is large, and we shall be dealing in detail with the most common reactions to illness (and how to respond to them) in chapter 5. For the present, it is important to be aware of the very wide range of individual fears and concerns that patients may express about illness (and hence bad news). From the professional's point of view, the only safe assumption is that one can safely assume nothing.

Furthermore, it is not always easy to estimate the impact of an illness on a patient from our own knowledge of that particular illness. What, as a health care professional, you might regard as a trivial illness (such as genital herpes), because it is not life-threatening, might be devastating to the patient because of the threat it poses to his or her hopes, ambitions, expectations, or social standing. Conversely, occasionally a patient accepts with calm an illness that you thought would be overwhelming.

Hence, the impact on an individual patient can only be assessed in the context of that patient's life (mild osteoarthritic changes in the foot might not alter your life very much, but would radically

affect you if you happened to be a footballer or a ballet dancer).
It is obviously impractical and impossible for every professional
to get into every single patient's life sufficiently to assess the impact
of every medical diagnosis you make. We are not required to live
every person's life in order to be her or his physician or nurse,
even if it were possible. However, as part of the technique of
breaking bad news, we can use an approach in which we gain a
better understanding of the impact of the illness on the patient.
This is the major advantage of the second and third steps of the
protocol that follows in chapter 4.

> **Ground Rule: When it comes to anticipating a patient's
> reaction, there is only one safe assumption – it is not safe
> to assume anything!**

DOCTOR FACTORS

As health care professionals (whether we are doctors, nurses, or
members of any other discipline) we are subject to various sources
of pressure that make the interview uncomfortable for us. Some
of these stem from the fact that we are human beings (albeit
professionals) in a room with other human beings (patients) who
are in distress. Other sources of pressure start during, or are amplified by, our professional training.

Fear of causing pain

Bad news causes pain to the person hearing it, and as health care
professionals we naturally find the act of inflicting pain unpleasant. Furthermore, in most of our training we are taught to relieve
pain, and if it is necessary that we inflict it (during surgery for
example), we are accustomed to giving an anaesthetic or analgesic
to minimize or remove it. Unfortunately, there can be no anaesthetic that removes the pain of hearing bad news – the patient
has to be awake and mentally competent in order to understand
the situation. For us to consciously inflict pain on a conscious
patient seems to upset the normal rules of our relationship with
the patient, and is one reason we often try to avoid it.

Sympathetic pain

We are also quite likely to experience considerable discomfort sim- ply by being in the same room as someone who is going through the distress caused by bad news. This sympathetic pain may seem such a simple and obvious idea that it does not need to be stated, but even so in our professional practice we often feel uncomfort- able and distressed and may not realize in the heat of the moment that our distress originates with the patient's distress. We are there- fore experiencing no more than (and no less than) the sympathetic counterpart of the patient's experience.

In addition to the social and sympathetic reasons for finding the interview difficult, there are additional factors that are introduced or amplified during professional training (particularly medical school). These additional factors are created inadvertently as by- products – side effects, perhaps – of medical training, but even though they are accidental, they still increase the difficulty of breaking bad news, and are detailed in the following paragraphs.

Fear of being blamed

There are two elements to our fear of being blamed. The first is caused by the basic human characteristic of blaming the messenger for the bad news that he or she brings. The second is the feeling imbued into us during our training that when a person's health deteriorates there must be somebody at fault (an attitude that is strongly reinforced by medico-legal practices).

Blaming the messenger for the bad news: Humankind does not seem to be very good at dealing with bad news in the abstract. Intellectually, humans find it very difficult to grasp and grapple with bad news when it arrives, and people have a great propensity to personify the bad news, to identify it with another person (usu- ally the person who bring it), and thus to direct their sense of anger or outrage at that person.

To take an example from daily life, think of what happens when someone parks his or her car illegally and then comes back to find an officer writing out a parking ticket. The motorist is extremely unlikely to say something like *Well, officer, you're just doing your job. I suppose this is what I deserve for parking illegally.* In almost every instance, the motorist finds some reason, however spurious, for blaming this particular person (*Couldn't you see I was just shopping for my kids* or *You're enjoying this aren't you – it's because I've got a Volvo and you haven't*). In fact, it is even easier to blame the officer for the ticket because the officer wears a uniform, and one is therefore directing one's anger and resentment not at Mr. Joe Soap who has a family of his own and is quite nice when you get to know him, but, through the uniform of Officer J. Soap, at the majesty of the Parking Ticket Department and at the faceless and nameless bureaucrats whose lives are devoted to upsetting ours.

If the example seems slightly frivolous, the underlying behavior is not. This is the way in which human beings tend to react to bad news. They blame the messenger for the bad news, and find it easier to do so if the messenger carries a badge of authority that slightly depersonalizes him or her. We all react in this way and we all know we do, so that when, as health care professionals, it is our turn to break the bad news (wearing our uniforms and carrying our badges of office), we quite rightly fear the blame that accompanies the duty.

In fact, many of the outward symbols of the health care professional that are so useful in supporting the patient draw blame towards us when the news is bad. We are perceived as having a great deal of control over our patients' lives (we tell them when they need tests, when they need to go to hospital, when they can leave, and so on), we enjoy professional privilege (including access to the intimate details of our patient's lives and anatomies) and social status (including a good income). All these things are seen as setting the professional apart from the lay person, and are important (to varying degrees) in the professional relationship, because to some extent they depersonalize us and allow the patient to feel that he or she is dealing with the mainstream of medical science not just an ordinary person with a stethoscope or a thermometer.

However, when the news is bad and the patient perceives medical science as failing him or her, these outward symbols of authority may attract even more blame. The professionals are seen as taking the credit for any triumphs and therefore are the justifiable targets for blame if there are defeats. We are the ones who bring the news and are thus perceived as the ones responsible for it, and most of our professional manners and trappings accidentally line us up as the main targets for the patient's feelings of anger and resentment.

Fear of therapeutic failure: As professionals, we add further fuel to that human desire to blame the messenger by reinforcing the idea that all deterioration and death must be attributable to a failure of the medical system or the staff. This is not a deliberate stance, but is a side effect of the attitude that modern medicine has "a pill for every ill." Over the past few decades, the medical profession has entered into a reciprocating relationship with the general public that has fostered the illusion that all diseases are fixable. Inadvertently, we seem to be denying the idea that death is ultimately inevitable (although, as somebody once said, *despite all the best interventions of modern medicine, the death rate will always remain the same – precisely one per person*). We therefore allow (however passively) the mantle of omnipotence to rest on our shoulders.

Furthermore, our training in medical school reinforces this feeling (albeit inadvertently). In all our training we are taught (appropriately) to deal with the myriad of reversible or treatable conditions. Whether these conditions are common or rare, it is obviously important that future doctors and nurses should be able to treat the treatable ones. It is equally obvious that someone who fails to recognize and treat a potentially treatable condition is culpable. However, the curriculum is so full of these conditions that there is virtually no teaching on the subject of therapeutic impotence. What do you do when you cannot reverse the disease? The answer, of course, is embodied in the entire discipline of palliative-care medicine, in which the therapeutic endeavor is directed not at the disease but at the symptoms. However, most medical schools and nursing colleges do not teach palliative-care medicine in the undergraduate curriculum, and as a result most medical students evolve into physicians who are keen to treat the curable conditions, but have little training in what to do with chronic irreversible diseases.

This sense of therapeutic failure, which has its beginnings in social attitudes and professional training, is exacerbated yet further by the current medico-legal atmosphere.

Medico-legal issues: Medico-legal factors make the load heavier still. The medico-legal atmosphere is changing in all countries, but basically it is becoming easier (particularly in the United States) to attach the blame for any medical deterioration to the doctor or nurse. This contributes to (or perhaps reflects) society's view that all patients have an inalienable right to be cured of any condition, and if they do not achieve that objective it must be the fault of some human agency, and that there must be legal and financial recourse for the person who believes that he or she is the victim of such a failure. Again, there are no rights or wrongs about this; it simply means that the atmosphere in which we practice is changing and that it is increasingly difficult for patients and doctors to face facts calmly when they include inevitable deterioration or death.

Fear of the untaught
We also fear the breaking of bad news if we have not been shown how to do it properly. In all our professional training we learn to obtain our rewards for doing a particular task "properly," which means "by following conventional procedures." If we deviate from conventional guidelines we expect to (and usually do) end up in trouble. We are thus trained and programmed to avoid deviations from standard practice. In most respects, this attitude is based on sound principles. We need to be efficient at following protocols and procedures in order to treat reversible conditions and medical emergencies. If a patient is in diabetic coma, it would clearly be most undesirable to have the physician in charge experiment with insulin or potassium, or try to work out what to do from first principles. There are guidelines for the treatment of diabetic coma because these produce the best results as shown in documented clinical experience. Thus, when there is a reversible condition, society (including our own microsociety – the health care professions) demands that the doctor does it "by the book." In these circumstances we feel pleased when the outcome is success, and

we may also be reassured that no other person could have done better if the outcome is failure.

While this is the accepted and justifiable norm for any procedure for which there are guidelines, if there happen to be no guidelines – as in the case of breaking bad news – then we will naturally feel ill at ease and will show a tendency to avoid the matter entirely. We do not enjoy doing something if we have not been taught how to do it properly. This tendency almost always becomes worse as we increase our skills in other areas. The more competent we are at reading ECGs or interpreting chest X-rays, the more difficult it becomes to face up to the fact that we do not know how to do the apparently simple task of sitting down and just talking, because nobody has told us how to do it or how to know when we are doing it properly. It is therefore essential for professionals in any health care discipline to be as thoroughly trained in patient communication skills as they are in other clinical skills. Furthermore, if learning these skills is a compulsory part of the curriculum in medical schools and nursing colleges, they will also be perceived as being an essential component of clinical management. If they are excluded, they will be regarded as "optional," and clinicians will feel more and more uneasy about their own interviewing skills later on. Filling this gap in the syllabus is one of the main purposes of this book (and the video course on which it is based).

Fear of eliciting a reaction
In the same way in which, as professionals, we dislike doing tasks for which we have not been trained, so we also fear the side effects or reactions caused by any intervention unless we have been taught how to cope with them. This is another axiom of medical practice: "do not do anything unless you know what to do if it goes wrong." Again, this is perfectly reasonable – we do not attempt cystoscopy unless we know how to recognize and deal with a perforated bladder, and we do not even take a blood sample until we know what to do if we hit an artery. This training, however essential for daily practice, means that if nobody has taught us how to cope with a patient who cries or becomes angry, we will avoid any interview that might produce this "side effect." This is why chapter 5 of this book is so long – and important.

Furthermore, interviews in which patients show emotional reactions may earn discouraging responses from other professionals.
Although it is less common nowadays than a few years ago, there
are still senior physicians and senior nurses who think it is a bad
thing to "get the patient all upset." That kind of disapproval is
hard to deal with. If you have taken the trouble to talk to a patient
about something that is painful for him or her, it is very discouraging to be blamed for having caused the upset. It should be an
obvious fact (but it is often ignored) that if you have had an
interview about a patient's cancer diagnosis, and if the patient,
for example, bursts into tears, you have not caused the tears (the
cancer diagnosis is the central cause – see below). All you have
done is to cause the emotions to be expressed at that particular
time and in that particular place. In many respects it is both important and flattering that the patient has trusted you enough to
share his or her pain with you, and it is also important that the
patient feels confident enough to cry in front of you instead of
bottling it up and taking it all home. Unfortunately, doctors and
nurses (particularly if they are lower in the hierarchy) often do
get the blame for causing the upset, and disapproval is often expressed most strongly by staff members who themselves find this
situation uncomfortable.

Finally, there is the important point that choosing not to talk
about the diagnosis with the patient does not make the illness
disappear. While it may be true that a bad-news interview upsets
the patient, the subsequent impact of the illness will upset the
patient much more, and may be far greater if the patient is unprepared for it. A patient who finds out later that you had some
important information and chose not to give it may be far more
upset (as may his or her lawyers) than a patient hearing the bad
news when you first know about it. In other words, if serious
illness is upsetting for the patient, then you may not have the
option of protecting him or her from all distress. The illness is the
cause of the distress, not the interview.

To put it simply, if the patient's medical condition is going to
deteriorate, then your real choice is not between "upsetting the
patient" and "not upsetting the patient." The real choice is between "having the patient react to the illness and prepare for it

now" and "leaving the patient unprepared, and facing a bigger reaction later." If the chest X-ray is abnormal, your decision to hide the information from the patient will not unfortunately, turn the X-ray into a normal one.

Fear of saying "I don't know"

In our professional training we are never rewarded for saying *I don't know*. From our first days to our final examinations (and thereafter) we expect our standing to be diminished if we confess that we do not know all the answers. Perhaps it is one of the truest principles of communication with patients that "real life is not like your final exams." In real life (that is, communicating with real human beings called patients) honesty shown by a professional always strengthens the relationship, increases trust, and encourages honesty in return. Conversely, attempts to baffle or deceive the patient, or attempts to bluff by disguising ignorance or pretending greater knowledge or experience, will weaken the bond between the patient and professional and will discourage honest dialogue.

> **Ground Rule: Bluffing sometimes works in exams – but usually not in real life.**

Fear of expressing emotions

It is hardly surprising that professionals (particularly doctors) have difficulty in showing their emotions: most training curricula specifically proscribe it. There are good reasons for this. We have to remain calm in order to think clearly and logically, and certain emotions such as anger or panic damage our ability to make good clinical judgments. It is also a central rule of the code of our profession that we do not display emotions such as irritation or panic (as far as is humanly possible), since this is regarded as unprofessional behavior and weakens the trust that patients place in the profession as a whole. Suppressing the display of these emotions is therefore important for two reasons: decision-making and professional behavior.

However, while we are being trained not to show panic or rage, inadvertently we are also being encouraged to visualize the ideal professional as one who never shows any emotions at all and is consistently unflappable and brave (along the lines of a John Wayne or Clint Eastwood super-hero). Maintaining this image leaves us unprepared for a bad-news interview. When we break bad news, our patients expect us to have feelings of our own, and we will appear to be cold-hearted and indifferent if we do not know how to deal with them. Our own emotions (unless antagonistic or hostile) can become a valuable part of our support of the patient, provided that we know how to recognize and use them appropriately. If we have not been taught how to deal with, express, and exploit our own emotions to help the patient, we will try to suppress or disguise them. In doing so we will unwittingly increase the distance between ourselves and the patient. As we shall see in the next chapter, we are not required to cry or bleed for every one of our patients, but very often our ignorance about which emotions are "allowed" or "permissible" in a doctor-patient relationship stifles even the simplest expressions of human sympathy and support.

In fact, our professional training and authority make it even more difficult for us in this respect than for nonprofessionals. In our course at the University of Toronto, we ask the medical students what they would do if one evening the next-door neighbor knocked on the door and said *My doctor says I have cancer*. Most medical students know what they would do: invite the neighbor in, make tea, express sympathy, listen to the neighbor talking, and so on. Unfortunately, when those same students put on their white coats and try to deal with the same situation in a clinical setting, they often do not know what to do. In part this is due to the misconception that doctors ought to know what to say on every occasion, and that somehow medical support ought to be different from ordinary human "next-door-neighbor" support. Since the student hasn't been told what to do in this circumstance and therefore does not know whether his or her own emotions are "permitted" or not, he or she may be unable to use even the basic human resources and vocabulary that would otherwise be available.

Furthermore, even if we want to show some human sympathy,

the moment we start to do so there are some linguistic problems that threaten to trip us up.

Ambiguity of the phrase "I'm sorry": Most of us forget that the word "sorry" has two quite distinct meanings. It can be a form of sympathy (*I am sorry for you*) and can also be a form of apology, accepting responsibility for an action (*I am sorry that I did this*). Unfortunately, both are customarily abbreviated to *I'm sorry*. In fact, the ambiguity is so deeply ingrained that when the word is used in its rarer sense (of conveying sympathy) it is often misunderstood. Conversations like this are not rare:

> A: ... and then my mother was brought into hospital.
> B: Oh, I'm sorry.
> A: You've got nothing to be sorry for.

The first speaker is so used to hearing the word "sorry" as an apology that she or he responds with a reflex reply to an apology before realizing that it was not an apology that was being offered, but an expression of sympathy.

This has relevance to us as professionals. Not only is it difficult for us to overcome some of our trained responses in order to express our own human emotions of sympathy and empathy, but the moment we try to do so, we fall foul of this linguistic slip and appear to be accepting responsibility (with the associated medico-legal implications) instead of offering support.

The solution to this ambiguity lies in paying careful attention to you own speech patterns. It is not difficult to make sure that if you intend to say I am sorry you take care to use the specific words I am sorry for you. There are, however, better ways of expressing an empathic response, and in chapter 5 we shall be exploring different ways of expressing support with only occasional use of the word "sorry."

Fear of one's own illness/death

Most of us – if we ever think of these subjects in personal terms – have some degree of fear about serious illness or about our own death. In fact, some psychologists suggest that every health care professional's desire to be a doctor or nurse is partly based on a desire to deny one's own mortality and vulnerability to illness. This is sometimes called counterphobic behavior, and in real terms it means that each time we enter into an encounter with a sick person and, as it were, walk away from the encounter unharmed, we are reinforcing our own illusions of immortality and invulnerability.

It is difficult to estimate how important this fear is for each individual. However, most professionals probably are to some extent afraid of illness and death, and this might make it difficult to get emotionally attached to patients, particularly if we perceive them as similar to ourselves. Identifying with a patient makes it easy to think *There, but for fortune, go I* – which in turn challenges the invisible line that we may have drawn between Us (as health care professionals) and Them (as patients).[19] This attitude may or may not be important in any individual professional, but there are obvious instances where a physician finds it extremely uncomfortable to deal with a patient who seems to resemble himself or herself, or perhaps a parent, child, or sibling.

The value of this present exercise is in helping identify the components of your own discomfort when you experience it. If you are able to see that your desire to avoid a particular situation is partly based on motives such as this one, you will be better able to compensate for that tendency.

Fear of the medical hierarchy

Finally, in this list of things that make it difficult for us to discuss bad news, we have to face the fact that we live in the real world. In the real world, not all professionals think of these issues as important (perhaps because of their own fears of illness and death, or fears of the untaught, and so on). This means that if you are a junior member of a team, occasionally you will be under pressure from a senior staff member when you try to discuss bad news. In more old-fashioned hierarchical systems (in Britain in the sixties, for instance) it was quite possible for senior physicians to say something such as *no patient of mine is ever to be told that they have cancer*. Nowadays that stance is less tenable for ethical and legal reasons, but you may still run into vestigial emotional reactions of the same type, and you may find it very difficult to respond to the patient's desire for information and support if it seems that you have to contravene somebody else's rulings to do so. Fortunately, there is a way out of this (as we shall see in chapter 6), since in any circumstances, however adverse, you can always perform advocacy and transmit the patient's questions and reactions and knowledge (or suspicions) upwards to the senior person concerned.

A greater difficulty: Facing death

So far, then, we have seen how the bad news itself causes discomfort to the patient and to the professional. Even though on most occasions the bad news that you will have to share with patients does not contain an implicit threat of dying, when it does it raises the intensity of the interview considerably and increases the difficulty for both you and the patient. There are many reasons for this, and it is worthwhile spending some time considering the causes of that discomfort. We shall deal with these causes under the headings of social attitudes and patients' fears. We will then review the transition through which patients go as they face the end of life and will suggest a practical method of understanding that process.

SOCIAL ATTITUDES TO DYING

Contemporary society is going through a phase of virtual denial of death. Such things are probably cyclical, and we may now be seeing this denial phase beginning to fade. However, at present the subjects of death and dying are frequently termed "the ultimate obscenity" and "the last taboo," reflecting, at the very least, the difficulty our society has in talking about dying. Again, the price of this denial is paid by the person whose life is threatened and who has to face death, and also by us, as professionals, when we have to inform him or her of that threat. The major social roots of the fear of dying have been detailed elsewhere,[20] but to reiterate them briefly:

Lack of experience of death in family: Nowadays, most adults have not seen anyone die at home when they themselves were young and impressionable. This is in sharp contrast with the situation a century or so ago.

First, for centuries most Western families cohabited as extended families (which simply means that when a couple have children they remain living with their parents so that grandchildren and grandparents cohabit). The current pattern of the nuclear family (in which children move away when, or before, they become parents themselves) is relatively recent. Second, until the last four or five decades most deaths occurred at home (over 95 percent in Victorian times), whereas now the majority of deaths occur in a hospital or institution.

This means that most people who are now adult have not seen a relative die at home when they themselves were children, whereas a few decades ago most people would have had that experience. This is not to say that witnessing a death at home was necessarily a pleasant event, but simply that a child growing up as part of an extended family fifty years ago would be imprinted with a sense of the continuity of life, the process of aging, and the natural inevitability of dying ("when you are older you will look like dad, when you are much older you will look like granddad, when you are very very old you will die"). With the disappearance of the extended family and with dying becoming the province of the doctor and/or institution, most people have lost that sense of continuity and now regard the process of dying as something intrinsically alien and divorced from the business of living.

High expectations of health and life: Advances in medical science are often overreported in the media as "major breakthroughs." The constant bombardment of the public with the news of miraculous advances in the fight against disease subconsciously raises expectations for health and offers tantalizing hopes of immortality. This in turn makes it even harder for an individual to face the fact that he or she personally cannot be cured even though "They" could produce the miracles seen on television or in the papers. Again, the fascination with medical science and health is neither a good nor a bad thing; it is merely an attitude that has a price, and the price is paid by the individuals facing death and by those trying to support them.

Materialism: It might seem beyond the scope of a clinical textbook to assess the materialist values of the modern world, but it is relevant to the task of breaking bad news. Our society routinely evaluates a person's worth in terms of material and tangible values. If you ask someone *What kind of person is David?* you expect to hear something about his job, his rank or position, his accomplishments, and perhaps his home and family. You would be surprised to hear a non-material answer referring to his belief systems, such as *David – he's an existentialist.* In daily life we accept the material-based scale of appraisal without comment – it is the norm (and this is not the place for a pronouncement on whether that is good or bad). However, the one thing we all know about death (or most of us do, anyway) is that dying means being parted from material possessions. Hence, a society that places a high and almost exclusive value on material possessions again increases the price of dying for its members, and for those looking after them.

The changing role of religion: Without attempting a major theological analysis of our society, it can be fairly stated that the role of religion has changed, and that the commonly held view of a single, exterior, anthropomorphic God is now fragmented and individualized. Religion is currently much more of an individual philosophical stance than it was in the last century, and it is no longer possible to assume that everyone shares the same idea of a God and of an afterlife. A Victorian physician could say to a patient *Your soul will be with your Maker by the ebb tide* and genuinely mean that as a statement of fact and of consolation. Nowadays we cannot assume that a statement like that will bring relief to all, or even most, patients. Religion is still important to many people, but being more individualized, it is not readily accessible as a means of support to most of us who are not clerics.

For all these reasons, then, our society seems to be passing through a phase of development during which the process of dying is perceived as alien and fearsome, and during which the dying person is increasingly separated and divided from the living. This raises the discomfort that surrounds any conversation about dying – a particular, but not rare, example of the breaking-bad-news interview. However, in addition to the social reasons for this discomfort, there are personal ones as well.

PATIENTS' FEARS OF DYING

The fear of terminal illness and dying is far from being a monolithic emotional state. It can comprise hundreds of individuals fears. It is probably true to say that every human being will have a different and unique combination of fears and concerns. We will see how to elicit and respond to these individual fears in later chapters, but to illustrate the many varieties that exist, some of the major categories are set out in the following table.

COMMON FEARS ABOUT TERMINAL ILLNESS AND DYING

Fears about physical illness
physical symptoms (pain, nausea, etc.), disability (paralysis, loss of mobility)

Fears about psychological effects
not coping, "breakdown," losing one's mind/dementia, losing control

Fears about death
existential fears, religious concerns

Fears about treatment
side effects (baldness, pain), surgery (pain, mutilation), altered body image (surgery, colostomy, mastectomy)

Fears about family and friends
loss of sexual attraction or function, being a burden, loss of family role

Fears about finances, social status, and job
loss of job/power/status (as breadwinner), possible loss of medical insurance with job, treatment expenses, being "out of the mainstream"

At this point it is only important to note that fears about dying are not universal in nature, but are individual. As we shall see in chapter 5, your approach to the fears of dying should make no assumptions about which aspect is most important to the individual patient, but should elicit from the patient those aspects that she or he is particularly afraid of.

THE THREE-STAGE MODEL OF THE PROCESS OF DYING

Granted that our society in general, and the patient in particular, experiences considerable discomfort around the subject of dying, it is appropriate for us to discuss now the process of dying as we see it while looking after a patient from the earliest stage (the moment at which the patient first becomes aware of the possibility of dying as a personal reality, as opposed to an intellectual abstraction) onwards.[21]

A great deal has been written about the stages of dying, and several conceptual frameworks have been put forward, the best known being that of Dr. Elisabeth Kubler-Ross.[22] Her studies broke new ground in understanding the process of dying. She classified the process into five stages and termed them denial, anger, bargaining, depression, and acceptance. This model gained rapid and widespread acceptance within the health care professions and with the general public, and has been used and taught all over the world.

However, although this was unequivocally important and new work, there have been many difficulties in applying this framework to the practical care of patients facing death. In particular, the system does not often "fit the bill" in terms of what happens in clinical practice, and frequently does not assist the professional in predicting what is likely to happen next, or by what criteria he or she can assess the patient's reactions.

The most significant deficiency of the system is, first, that the five stages are important and common *reactions* to the threat of death, but not (with the exception of acceptance) true *stages* of dying. Second, human beings do not experience emotions in serial stages, but have their own mixtures of emotions together and simultaneously. It is worth spending a little time considering these aspects, since they are crucial to the understanding of patients' responses to the threat of dying, and therefore are crucial to any interview about bad news in which the threat of dying is perceived by the patient.

Reactions vs stages

Confronted with a serious threat such as death, an individual exhibits reactions that are characteristic of that person and of the way in which she or he has reacted to difficulties in the past, not of the stage in the process or the diagnosis. In other words, the emotions that the patient displays tell the observer something about the person, not about the stage that he or she is passing through. We all develop our own inbuilt repertoire of emotions as we grow up (subject presumably to our experiences in childhood and other factors). Some people are easily roused to anger and others are not; some greet every reverse or trouble by turning their backs and shutting it out, while other face it directly and wish to know the worst possible outcome as early as they can; some are eager to please and find it difficult to live with unresolved confrontation, while others have no difficulty in functioning in such an atmosphere; and so on. Each of us carries around our personal internal palette of emotions from which we pick our own emotional reactions. These reactions are, thus, better thought of not as stages of a universal process but as the essential components of the emotional side of each person's character.

Simultaneous vs serial emotions

If we think about the way human beings experience emotions, it seems more realistic to think of them as experienced simultaneously rather than serially. Think, for example, of what happens when a parent loses a child temporarily in a supermarket and then finds the child again. At that instant, the parent experiences relief, guilt, happiness, anger (at both child and self), fear (over what might have happened), and regret – all at the same time. These are not stages; they coexist and are contemporary with each other.

This illustration is an important analogy to what happens in facing the prospect of dying. For instance, denial and anger are often experienced at the same tie.   A patient may easily be angry with the disease but may express the anger as resentment at the doctor, while simultaneously exhibiting denial (in, for instance, accusing the doctor of making a mistake in the diagnosis). Intellectually, these emotions are incompatible (how can you be angry at something whose very existence you are denying?), but emotionally they frequently coexist. This is simply the way the human mind works, and it is more useful to think of human beings as mosaics rather than chameleons.

Reactions missing from the five-stage model

There are also common features of patients' reactions to dying that are missing from the five-stage model. The first, and most obvious, is fear. Fear of dying is so universal[23] that if a particular patient does not exhibit it, one's first thought should be *Has this patient understood the situation?* There are the exceptional individuals who are so comfortable and well-balanced in their lives that they can face the end of life with perfect equanimity. However, such people are rare, and one would be advised to first exclude misunderstanding (conscious or subconscious) as an explanation for the absence of fear. Certainly, any attempt to describe the process of dying should include some mention of fear within the model.

Second, there is guilt, which is a very common reaction to dying (and will be considered in detail in chapter 5) and is seen so often that it too should be accommodated in any conceptual framework that relates to the clinical picture. Third, it seems that hope and despair tend to alternate with each other on a cyclical basis, and it is extremely difficult to "track" the patient unless you realize that hope and despair are alternative emotional responses to the same facts. Furthermore, many patients use humor as a copying strategy to maintain a sense of perspective in the face of potentially overwhelming news, and this too requires a place in any conceptual framework.

False entities

It also seems quite likely that bargaining is not a stage that most patients go through, but an attempt at intellectualization used by certain individuals in order to provide a rational link between the worst-case scenario that they fear and the best-case scenario that they hope for. In other words, bargaining appears to be, not a stage per se, but an individual coping strategy.

The three-stage model (beginning–middle–end)
For all these reasons, it seems that the process of dying is not
accurately described by the five-stage model. In the broadest view,
it seems that in facing death, an individual makes a transition from
"ordinary life" (with its inherent illusion of immortality) to the
acceptance (if it is reached) of death as imminent and inevitable.
That transition can be thought of as a progression from normal
life (which can be characterized as *I know that I'll die some day but
usually behave as if I won't*) to the beginning stage of dying (*I now
realize that I might die of this particular disease*) to the middle stage
(*I realize that I will die of this particular disease but am not dying
now*) to the final stage (*I am dying*).

   As the patient makes this progression (whether or not he or she
reaches the final stage of fully accepting that death is imminent),
the reactions that you – as a professional – will see are typical,
not of the stage, but of the patient and that patient's coping strategies. This conceptual framework seems a much more logical and
practical method of thinking about the process of dying, and is
summarized in the following table.

THE THREE-STAGE MODEL OF THE PROCESS OF DYING

Initial stage *Facing the threat*	Chronic stage *Being ill*	Final stage *Acceptance*
A mixture of reactions that are characteristic of the individual and may include any or all of: Fear Anxiety Shock Disbelief Anger Denial Guilt Humor Hope/despair Bargaining	1 Resolution of those elements of the initial response that are resolvable 2 Diminution of intensity of all emotions ("monochrome state") 3 Depression is very common.	1 Defined by the patient's acceptance of death 2 Not an essential state provided that patient is not distressed, is communicating normally, and is making decisions normally

Initial stage – "Facing the threat": As the patient first appreciates the threat to life as a reality, he or she exhibits reactions that are often acute and intense, and that are characteristic of that person's reactions to stress (angry people get angry, people who habitually use denial will use a lot of denial, and so on). What you see as a professional is, therefore, a miniature portrait of the patient. If you had had access to the patient's life at crucial moments in the past (for instance, in failing to get a promotion, in marital difficulties or whatever) you would have seen the same kind of responses, the same patterns of reaction.

The significance of understanding and recognizing those reactions in the initial ("facing the threat") stage is that you will not see them change in nature, but will see them be resolved (if they can, with assistance) and diminish in intensity as the patient progresses. In the first section of chapter 5 we will review the patient's reactions and assess how to decide whether a particular reaction is assisting the patient or not, and whether or not, if a reaction is not helping the patient, the situation can be remedied.

Chronic stage – "Being ill": The middle or chronic ("being ill") stage of dying is the one in which patients are often "living with the prospect of dying." It is the stage in which the patient knows (overtly or subliminally) that recovery is not possible, but is not in danger of imminent death. This phase is characterized by a form of coexistence between the patient and the threat of dying. Those parts of the acute reactions that are resolvable have been resolved – the emotional colors are the same but their intensity is diminished.

For a few patients, this phase does not exist. Some patients are incapable, even with assistance, of resolving the intensity of their emotional responses and remain, as it were, at full throttle right to the end of life. For most, however, some or all of the initial reactions fade, and the peaks and valleys of emotional intensity are smoothed out. However, the patient's life – if apparently calmer – is often far from normal. If there is a single emotion seen commonly in the "being ill" stage it is depression. Often, once the acute phase is over the drama departs, and the family and friends depart with it. This is not to say that support commonly disappears entirely, but often once the fluster and flurry is reduced the patient is alone for more of the time. This chronic phase is often tiresome and boring for patient and family, and it is during this time that the health care professionals should be particularly on the alert.

Final stage – "Acceptance": The final phase – in this system as in that of Kubler-Ross – is defined by the acceptance of death by the patient. However, many practitioners (the authors of this book included) would suggest that although acceptance is useful and occurs in the majority of cases, not every patient needs to accept death overtly in order to face death "normally." If the patient is free of distress, is communicating normally with friends and family, and is making informed decisions in a way that is appropriate for him or her, then many professionals would suggest that that person is facing death in a perfectly satisfactory manner, even if there is no overt acceptance of it. However, this situation is not common and should be diagnosed only after the professional has made a serious attempt to detect any hidden distress that the patient may be feeling. Then, if those signs are absent – even if the patient shows no overt acknowledgment of death – he or she may be supported in that state without a forced acceptance of death.

If you find that the three-stage system proposed here allows you to conceptualize your patients' experiences and to recognize and predict their behavior, then that – to some extent – validates the framework as a practical guide to this awkward and difficult area. We shall be demonstrating approaches to the various emotional responses in chapter 5, which deals with general approaches to emotional reactions in the first part, and specific reactions in the second.

SUMMARY

1   Bad news is any news that drastically and negatively alters the patient's view of her or his future. The "badness" of bad news is the gap between the patient's expectations and the medical reality.

2   Bad news about health brings into play social stigmata
        that exist before the patient comes to the doctor.

3   Patients fear bad news for many reasons, as do doctors
        (partly for the same reasons, partly for additional reasons
        reinforced by professional training).

4   All of these problems are made worse if the bad news
        carries with it the threat of dying.

5   The process of dying is a three-stage one during which
        each individual expresses emotions and responses that are
        characteristic of that person, not the stage. Several differ-
        ent emotions may be expressed simultaneously.

FURTHER READING

Becker E. The denial of death. New York: Free Press, 1973
Buckman R. I don't know what to say. London: Macmillan, 1988
Glaser BG, Strauss AL. Awareness of dying. New York: Aldine Publishing,
    1965
Kubler-Ross E. On death and dying. New York: Free Press, 1969
Maynard D. Breaking bad news in clinical settings

3 Basic Communication Skills

Professional listening

The purpose of this chapter is to emphasize the techniques necessary to demonstrate that you are actually listening to your patient. Much of this material may be familiar (particularly if you have had training in medical interviewing skills), but it rarely does harm to refresh your memory.

Occasionally professionals will seem (to our patients) to be extremely bad at listening. In most cases we are somewhat better at listening than we appear to be, but are perceived as being bad at it because we are not paying attention to the rules of good listening. These rules are not particularly complex, but they are not followed (or even necessary) in most of our everyday life and therefore do not come naturally to us when we need them.

In many situations of daily life we can get by with only brief or monosyllabic responses as signs that we are listening (occasionally we can get by with none at all, using actions alone) without causing major offense. (One favourite example of apparently inattentive listening is the old comedy sketch in which a wife talks for some minutes to her husband who is hidden behind his newspaper; when she says *Jack, are you listening to me?* he wearily lays aside his paper and gives a three-word summary of each of the topics that she has mentioned. This illustrates, among other things, the frustration that people feel when they think they are not being heard, as well as the low standards of listening in daily life – or at least in the daily life portrayed in situation comedies.) As emotional temperatures rise, however, it becomes more important to show that the speaker is being heard.

Why patients are unhappy

In clinical practice, too, the biggest problems are caused by not showing that you are listening to your patient, and patients' dissatisfaction with their doctors' communication skills far outweighs any dissatisfaction with technical competence.[24] Obviously some of the unhappiness is caused by what they are hearing, but dissatisfaction with the way that they hear it is most commonly caused by
- the doctor not listening or not appearing to listen,[25]
- the doctor using jargon, or
- the doctor talking down to the patient.

Let us look at these problems in greater detail and then consider some of the ways of improving listening skills to avoid these pitfalls.

Doctors not listening to their patients: As physicians one of the commonest misdemeanours that we commit is simply not letting the patient talk. Detailed studies[26] of doctors' interviews with patients reveal some rather upsetting statistics. Patients in a general-medicine setting attend with between 1.2 and 3.9 major complaints. On average, the time that the patient is allowed to talk before being interrupted by the physician is eighteen seconds, and only 23 percent of patients ever finish their opening statements. It is salutary to note two other points: (1) the first complaint that a patient mentions may not be the most important and (2) even if allowed to talk without interruption, the patient usually talks for no longer than 150 seconds (so by interrupting you're probably only saving 132 seconds anyway!).

Fortunately, the remedy is not very difficult – effective listening does improve patients' satisfaction with their doctors,[27] particularly if they are allowed to tell their own story in their own words[28] and express their feelings.[29] It also increases the perceived competence of the physician,[30] as well as enhancing the patient's compliance with the doctor's treatment plan.[31] (Later in this section we will illustrate techniques of demonstrating that you have listened to and heard what the patient has said.)

> **Ground Rule: "Let the people speak!" Then show you've heard.**

Doctor using medical jargon: When we do speak to patients we have a tendency to use what the patients regard as jargon. Of course, to us it is a highly efficient language and a way of transmitting precise (sometimes) information in a short time. To the patient it is an unintelligible language that doctors hide behind in order to avoid the pain of telling bad news or other painful or worrying information. Studies show that jargon confuses and alienates the patients, often leading to misunderstanding[32] and misinterpretation.[33] In fact, just over half of our patients will misunderstand significant portions of what we say,[34] and on average, 50 per cent of what is said is forgotten.[35] (The value of plain English over "medspeak" will be reinforced later in chapter 4.)

Doctors talking down to their patients: Another major cause of communication difficulty is the fact that we often patronize our patients, and talk down to them.[35] It has to be said that not all patients want communication on an equal level. In fact, the patient's pre-existing belief about the ideal physician-patient relationship may have a major effect on satisfaction in this area. Some patients want an authoritative figure, while the doctor wants an egalitarian sharing relationship. Other patients want the doctor to represent the parent they never had, while the doctor wants to behave as a scientist. Still other patients want no more than the practitioner's technical skills, while the doctor wants to become involved with the patient-as-person.[37] And so on. In all events, the doctor has to be sensitive to the fact that patronization is a common temptation[38] and that some of her or his patients may want different types of doctor-patient relationships. When it comes to communication there is no "one size fits all."

The best way for a doctor to avoid crossed transactions is to try as much as possible to talk to patients as equals (since that is what the majority of patients want). If the patient wishes the doctor to assume the one-up position and dominate the relationship (especially common with elderly patients[39]), the patient may indicate this (*You tell me what to do, doctor, I can't decide* or *You know what is best for me, doctor*). It is helpful to be able to detect the signals and have the flexibility in your style to assume the more authoritative position.[40]

The basic steps of the medical interview

There is a basic structure to dialogue between a patient and a health-care professional. It is not particularly complex, but unfortunately most of us are never told what it is, and so may fall short of the patient's expectations without realizing it. In essence the structure is as follows:

- Preparing for listening
- Questioning
- Listening actively
- Showing that you've heard
- Responding

The rest of this chapter will focus on guidelines that will help all medical interviews to proceed as efficiently and satisfactorily (for both parties) as possible. Then, in chapter 4, we will illustrate the additional structuring that makes up the protocol for breaking bad news.

PREPARING FOR LISTENING

All clinical interviews contain the potential for going wrong, and very often the seeds of dissatisfaction are sown in the first few minutes. When you start any clinical interview (which is always an unknown quantity and may contain all manner of unpleasant surprises for the patient or for you), it is worth spending a few

seconds getting the setting and the physical context right to minimize any discomfort (on your part or the patient's). A lot of this
is no more than courtesy and good manners, but if you don't do
it you will appear to be discourteous and to have bad manners.
A little bit of extra effort here pays dividends later on.

To make these guidelines easier to follow, we shall consider
them in the order in which the professional usually carries out a
clinical interview.

Introductions

Before you start any interview, check that the patient knows who
you are and what you do. Obviously if you are seeing the patient
regularly that is unnecessary, but occasionally we are so keen to
get on with the interview with a patient we have met only once
(or not at all) that we forget the introductions. This should not
happen.

If you are meeting the patient for the first time, most professionals suggest that you use the patient's surname unless invited
by the patient to use the first name. This depends on the age and
comfort level of the patient (and you), but you are much less likely
to cause offense if you start with "Mrs. Smith" and move on to
"Nancy" by invitation than if you start with "Nancy" and get a
frosty reception. Having introduced yourself, explain in three or
four words what you do. (If you're a medical student, say so:
everybody know what medical students are, and that all doctors
were students once.)

The handshake

As part of the introduction, if you are a physician or medical
student, it may be worth starting each interview by shaking hands
with the patient. (For some arbitrary reason, this is not necessarily
part of the behaviour that patients expect from certain professionals, such as nurses, or in certain clinical settings, such as busy
emergency departments.) If you can get into the habit of doing
that, and do it naturally and comfortably, you will find that it
reduces tension at the outset of the interview. It is, of course, a
personal touch (literally), and requires a certain commitment to
intimacy on the part of both participants. It is, therefore, one way
of telling the patient that you are (at least partly) a human being.

Practice Point: As a matter of observation, the handshake often tells you something about the family dynamics as well. Frequently the patient's spouse will extend his (or her) hand as well. It is always worth making sure that you shake the patient's hand before the spouse's – even if the spouse is physically nearer to you. In this way you demonstrate that the patient comes first, and the spouse – although an important member of the team – comes second.

Obviously, if you are at an early point in your career, you might be a little uncomfortable with shaking the patient's hand at first, but it is worth persevering with the practice until you feel comfortable. A little gesture with which you feel comfortable early on in the interview goes a long way to setting the patient at ease.

Having observed some common courtesies, you should then make sure the physical context of the interview is as conducive as possible to easy communication.

The physical context

In controlling the physical setting of the interview the first (and almost inviolable) rule (for all important communications by all health care professional disciplines) is **sit down**! Only if it is absolutely impossible to sit should you try and hold a significant clinical interview while standing (there are some hints about this in chapter 4). It doesn't matter what you sit on, be it your chair, the bed, a stool, or even a commode (which all too often is the only seat near the bedside in hospitals).

Practice Point: If the commode is the only seat, you should first ask if you may sit there – which will diminish any potential embarrassment. (As is the case with any potential cause of embarrassment, if you identify and acknowledge the factor of which you and the patient are both aware, you will markedly decrease its embarrassing effect.)

However you achieve it, sitting down sends important signals to the patient: that you are there to listen, that you are (to some extent) under the control of the patient, and (if your eyes are level with the patient's) that you would like to engage in non-patronizing communication. Furthermore, clinical anecdotes[41] suggest that when the doctor sits down, the patient perceives the length of time spent at the bedside as longer than if the doctor remains standing. (So, not only does the sitting down indicate to the patient that he or she has control and that you are there to listen, it saves you time as well.)

> **Ground Rule: When breaking bad news** *sit down* **(unless it is absolutely impossible to do so).**

Second, get any physical objects out of your way. Move any bedside tables, trays, or clutter out of the line between you and the patient. Ask for any televisions or radios to be turned off for a few minutes. If you are in an office or room, move your chair so that you are adjacent to the patient's not across the desk.

> **Practice Point:** If the physical act of rearranging the furniture causes you to feel awkward, you can state what you are trying to do (*Let's get this tray out of the way, so that we can talk freely* or *May we have the television turned off just for a moment so that we can concentrate?*).

Third, get the patient organized if necessary. If you have just finished examining the patient, allow (or assist) the patient to get dressed so that the sense of personal modesty can be restored.

Fourth, get yourself seated at a comfortable distance from the patient. This distance (sometimes called the "body buffer zone") seems to vary from culture to culture, but a distance of between twenty and thirty-six inches is suitable in American cultures for conversations about personal matters.[42] This is another reason why the doctor who remains standing at the end of the bed ("six feet away and three feet up," sometimes known as "the British position") seems remote and aloof.

The height you sit at can also be used to help you, and we will deal with that later, in chapter 5; however, for the moment assume that your normal position should be such that your eyes are approximately level with the patient's.

Your posture
Having got the physical context right, you should try and look relaxed – particularly if you do not feel relaxed (and few of us

do). To give yourself an air of relaxation, sit down comfortably with both your feet flat on the floor. Let your shoulders relax and drop. Undo your coat or jacket, if you are wearing one, to help emphasize the fact that you are not about to leave. Rest your hands on your knees. By and large, leaning back on the chair with one foot raised and crossed over the other leg (sometimes called "the open four" posture) will appear too casual and uninvolved for an interview that deals with bad news.

To touch – Yes or No?

Most medical schools do not teach specific details of touch at any time in the undergraduate curriculum,[43] which means that most of us have no specific guidelines on whether we should touch patients, or how. We are, therefore, likely to be ill-at-ease with touching as an interview technique until we have had some practice. Nevertheless, there is considerable evidence (although the data are somewhat "soft") that touching is of benefit during a medical interview (even though patients may not expect to be touched the first time they meet the physician[44]). If you have already shaken hands with the patient, to some extent the "touch-barrier" has already been broken – another advantage of starting the interview.

You should try to touch the patient at least once during the interview. If you are not comfortable doing it, watch other practitioners and see how (or if) they do it: a little emulation may increase your own abilities remarkably. During the more intense moments of the interview, a touch by a physician or nurse reduces the perceived emotional separation between you and the patient (as well as the physical distance). The most important part of the touch is to be sensitive to the patient's response. If the patient is comforted, continue; if the patient is uncomfortable, stop. Touch can be misinterpreted (as lasciviousness, aggression, or domination, for example), and it is often said that if there is any possibility of misinterpretation, you should avoid touching the patient below the waist (on the leg or knee) and limit any physical contact to the arm or shoulder. If you have not touched the patient at all during the interview, it is sometimes helpful to do this (a friendly touch on the arm, for instance) at the end.

Is this just fussiness?
All these details may seem somewhat fussy as you read them now,
and appear to be time-consuming. In practice they are not. It may
seem like a long time to get the setting right, but it only takes
twenty or thirty seconds and it saves many minutes of dissatisfaction (on both sides) later. However finicky it seems, this is the
point that starts the interview off on a stable course and sends an
immediate signal to the patient that you are in the role of a supporter. Doing all this will also make you feel more relaxed, because
you are following a pattern that is familiar to you and because
you have control of the messages you are sending to the patient.

QUESTIONING

A clinical interview is more than a mere conversation. It should
certainly include social dialogue and often may usefully encom-
pass some conversational elements, but it is much more than un-
directed or unfocused conversation. The clinical interview is a
specific (and often efficient) instrument by which information is
given by the patient and collected by the clinician, other information is transmitted to the patient, and opinions and emotions
are exchanged.
    Questioning is one of the fundamental tools of the interview,
and there are two major kinds of questions: open and closed.

Closed questions
Closed questions are ones that focus specifically on one particular
problem and offer the patient a limited number of answers – a
"yes" or "no" or else a multiple choice. Examples include all the
questions we use in history-taking (apart from the first open question *Tell me about the main problem that brought you here*). Examples
of closed questions include *Do you have swelling of the ankles?* (the
answer should be a yes or a no) or *How many times do you get up
to pass urine at night?* (the answer should be a number), and so
one. Closed questions are the staple of the medical history, and
an efficient method of gathering specific information quickly.
However, they do not give free range to the patients' interpretation
of events or to their ability to describe the events or their reactions

to them. Closed questions therefore prevent the discussion from moving on to any details or concerns of which the clinician is unaware, and has not asked about.

Open questions
Open questions are those that give the patient free rein to answer in any way she or he chooses. Examples include *How do you feel?*, *How did you react to that news?*, *What did you make of that chest pain?*, and so on. The essence of the open question is that it is does not force the patient to follow one particular train of thought in answering, nor does it define the focus of interest before the patient begins the answer. Obviously, open questions are not useful when you need specific detailed information on one aspect of the patient's problems, but they are extremely useful when you are opening up a new area of questioning, when you are investigating which direction to pursue in questioning, or when you do not have a clear understanding of what the patient felt or is feeling.

Biased questions (disguised statements)
Some sentences are phrased as questions but are not, in fact, questions at all. Biased questions are responses that we (occasionally) phrase in the form of a question, but which are statements about our assessment of the situation. They often reflect our own ambivalence – we know that we are under an obligation not to sit in judgment on a patient's situation but feel a strong desire to do so. In order to conform with what we see as professional behaviour, we disguise the judgment as a question. In this example,

> *Patient:* "... and my period's late so I think I'm pregnant."
> *Doctor:* "Don't you think it would be pretty careless for you to be pregnant while you haven't got a house or a job?"

the judgment is obvious (*pretty careless*), and the question (*Don't you think?*) is rhetorical. In breaking-bad-news interviews, as professionals we should always be aware of this tendency (in others and in ourselves), because a biased question often causes a sharp change in the atmosphere of the interview (usually by increasing hostility), and we may not realize what we have done to cause that change.

EFFECTIVE LISTENING (FACILITATING)

As the patient answers the questions, the listener has to show that she or he is in a listening mode. This is the basic skill of facilitation, and should, of course, be part of your repertoire for all interactions, not just breaking bad news. Here are the main guidelines.

Let the patient speak: If the patient is speaking, don't talk over him or her. Wait for the patient to stop speaking before you start your next sentence. This simplest rule of all is perhaps the most ignored, and its infringement the most likely to give the patient the impression that the doctor is not listening. Interruption should be avoided unless truly necessary to direct a talkative patient who is rambling.

> **Ground Rule: Only interrupt the patient if you absolutely have to.**

Encourage the patient to talk: You can use any or all of these: nodding, pauses, smiling, saying *Yes, Hmm hmm, Tell me more*, or anything similar. Maintain eye contact for most of the time while the patient is talking (sometimes if things are very intense, you can assist the patient by looking away briefly). Once you have completed the history-taking, try not to interrupt any subsequent exchanges by writing notes.

Tolerate short silences: If the patient falls silent, resist the temptation to fill the silence instantly. By and large, a patient will fall silent when he or she has feelings that are too intense to express in words. A silence usually means, therefore, that the patient is thinking or feeling something important, not that he or she has stopped thinking. If you can tolerate a pause or silence, the patient may well express the thought in words a moment later. If you have to break the silence, the ideal[45] way to do so is to say *What were you thinking about just then?* or *What is it that's making you pause?* or something to that effect.

> **Ground Rule: Silence is golden.**

Listen for the buried question: Patients are sometimes ambivalent about crucial questions: they may, for instance, want to ask a question, but only want to hear the answer if it's good news, and may fear the answer if it's not. Often the patient will reveal this ambivalence by burying the question – that is, asking the question in a soft voice while you are talking. This is not rare, and you should be on the alert for it. If the patient buries a question in this way, finish your sentence and then say something like *I'm sorry, you were about to ask me something*. Perhaps you should think of the buried question as a cause of patients not being listened to because they (partly) don't want to be listened to.

HEARING

Now the patient has started talking and you have been carefully listening. The next step is to show that you are *hearing* – and hearing is not quite the same as listening. "Hearing" implies that the listener has some measure of understanding, and that the speaker's words have some meaning. There are several mechanisms by which you can show that you have some understanding of the content of the patient's speech.

Repetition
Repetition is probably the single most important technique of all interviewing skills (apart from sitting down). To show that you are really hearing what the patient is saying, use one or two key words from the patient's last sentence in your first one. Here are two examples – one containing repetition, the other omitting it:

> *Patient:* ... and when I take the tablets three times a day, I feel sleepy.
> *Doctor:* Do you get nausea as well?
> *Patient:* ... and when I take the tablets three times a day, I feel sleepy.
> *Doctor:* The tablets make you feel sleepy?

In the first example the doctor is keen to find out whether it is the medication that is causing the drowsiness (a normal and appropriate objective). Since the medication also causes nausea he can find the answer quickly by asking about this other side effect. In doing so he has omitted to mention this missing linkage of medical facts to the patient and so has inadvertently given the impression to the patient that he regards the drowsiness as insignificant. This may or may not matter to the patient (depending on the situation): in the context of a routine medical interview it is probably not crucial, but in an interview about bad news, it may be that the doctor has missed an important opportunity to show that he or she is hearing the patient.

In the second example, the doctor indicated that he has heard about the drowsiness – he can then ask about nausea. His or her interview will take a few seconds longer, but at the end of it a major complaint (drowsiness) will have been given to the doctor, and will have been seen to be safely received. It is a little like registered mail – by the act of repetition, the doctor is signing the receipt showing that the message has been received by the addressee.

Repetition does not mean that you agree with what the patient has just said; it simply means that you have heard it. When the emotional temperature of the interview is high, hearing what the patient says is an important part of supporting the patient, but it does not imply professional endorsement of the patient's views.

Reiteration
Reiteration (often called paraphrasing) means repeating what the patient has told you but in your words, not hers or his. Your response in the example above might be *You seem to be getting some drowsiness from the tablets* (when the patient has used the word "sleepy"), and this would be a reiterative response.

Reflection
Reflection takes the act of listening one step further, and shows that you have heard and have interpreted what the patient said. (For example, *If I understand you correctly, you're telling me that you lose control of your waking and sleeping when you're on these tablets* ...) This is an important part of the interaction and will be illustrated further in the next section, but for the moment it should be noted that the foregoing are all techniques that enhance the professional's perceived ability as a listener.

RESPONDING

Thus far, then, we have a patient talking with a professional and receiving some indication that the words are being listened to, and heard. Obviously the professional's job does not stop with hearing (although it would be much simpler if it did): we have to respond to what we are hearing. However, although we have to respond we do not have to have all the answers to the patient's problems. In other words, our response must be sensitive to what the patient is expressing, but it does not have to show omniscience and omnipotence.

In formulating your response, you have several different options available to you. You can think of the options as specific tools in a toolbox that can be selected and used as the need arises. What follows are some guidelines that should help you decide which technique is going to advance the interview and maximize satisfaction (for the patient and, subsequently, yourself).

Further questions vs statements vs silence

For all the different emotions that it might contain, your response can be framed in only one of three ways. You can either ask further questions (in order to find out what is going on with greater accuracy) or you can make a statement (which reveals what you think is going on) or you can say nothing until the patient says something more. We have already detailed the difference between open and closed questions above; now the different types of statements can be examined. There are several methods of classifying responses. What follows is a combination of some of the simpler classifications.

Types of responses

Factual responses: Some questions are best answered by direct factual information. As professionals we are supposed to have a command of the relevant facts, or to be able to obtain the ones we do not immediately possess.

The aggressive/hostile response ("The counterattack"): Hostility expressed by patients is common, and if the disease appears to the patient to be serious, hostility is a frequent response. It is almost always an outward manifestation of fear, and originates with the patient's fear of the disease and anxieties about the future. Equally often it is manifested as anger towards those nearest – doctors, nurses, family, and friends. Unfortunately, as the target of hostility you cannot respond to it on the same level without seriously jeopardizing your professional relationship with the patient.

We shall be dealing with the details of how to respond to anger in chapter 5, but for the moment let us take a brief look at the way our response as a health care professional might be different from our response in ordinary life (if there is such a thing). In daily life we normally respond to aggression with an expression of our own aggression. This is quite normal and usually leads to escalation until one or other of the parties submits, or both parties resolve the issue or stop the dispute. In the medical interview, this type of attack – counterattack ("the hostile response") is almost always unproductive, and occasionally catastrophic.

In the medical interview, it is always best to attempt to see the root cause of the anger instead of responding to the manifestation itself. We shall see an example of how to do that in the last part of this section and again in chapter 5, but the principle is simple in theory (although far from easy in practice): it is to recognize the source of the anger, and not to respond to the display of anger, but to acknowledge the existence and origin of the emotion.

A hostile response to the displayed emotion, by contrast, erodes the professional nature of your relationship and makes all future communication insecure.

> *Scenario:* A patient has just been diagnosed as having lung cancer.
> *Patient says:* "I've got lung cancer and you're no damned use, you can't cure it."
> *Hostile response:* "Look, if you don't think I'm a good enough doctor, you're quite free to find yourself someone else."

This type of "take-it-or-leave-it" response would be perfectly normal (although clearly painful) in, for instance, a marital dispute. However, in the context of a doctor-patient relationship, it effectively closes the door and rules the doctor out as a means of support for the patient in the future. We shall look at other options at the end of this section.

The judgmental response: A judgmental response is the easiest to make and (often) the most difficult to resist. It is difficult to resist because "being judgmental" is one of the central functions of being a professional. We are constantly required to make clinical judgments, to distinguish the normal from the abnormal, and to propose interventions based on those judgments. It is actually difficult to stop doing that, which is why the judgmental response is so common and springs so readily to mind.

> *Scenario:* A patient has just been told that her cervical smear is positive (showing severe cervical dysplasia).
> *Patient says:* "Does my earlier sex life have anything to with my positive Pap test?"

Since cervical dysplasia is more common among those with early sexual exposure and with multiple partners, a factual response might be a simple one such as *Yes, it does,* whereas a judgmental response might be something such as *You can't lead a life of abandon and promiscuity with multiple partners and then expect that there isn't a price to be paid.* (However florid that may sound, it's taken from real life.)

> **Ground Rule: Hostile and judgmental responses come easily to hand – but they carry a high price later.**

The main problem with a judgmental response is that it is likely to stop dialogue unless the patient has asked for an evaluation or a judgment. In all other circumstances it closes lines of communication.

The reassuring response ("The pacifier"): The crucial element of a reassuring response is the attempt to decrease the patient's anxiety. There is nothing intrinsically wrong with this aim. The problem is that the reassuring response is often used automatically and early, before the patient's concerns have been heard. In those circumstances, it belittles the patient's feelings, and is perceived as a brush-off rather than a means of support.

> *Scenario:* The patient is a mother with mild lupus erythematosus, and early mild arthropathy.

56   How to Break Bad News

Patient says: "I'm very worried that I won't be able to take care
of my children."
Reassuring response: "Don't you worry about that sort of thing
– I'll do that kind of worrying about the future."

There is no criticism intended here of the physician's motivation.
The doctor clearly wants to assist the patient by reducing anxiety.
The problem with an early reassuring response (without acknowledging the existence of the patient's worry) is that it does not
produce that desired effect.

**Ground Rule: Premature reassurance – without
acknowledgment of the patient's feelings – doesn't reassure.**

The empathic response: The empathic response is one of the most
important ways in which you can respond to a patient's feelings,
but the phrase "empathic response" and its nature are frequently
misunderstood by medical students and others. The empathic response has three essential components, which are identifying the
emotion that the patient is experiencing, identifying the origins of
that emotion (in other words, the root causes of that emotion),
and responding in a way that tells the patient that you have made
those connections. It is a relatively simple interview technique, but
until it is formally demonstrated or taught it is usually overlooked
or ignored.

The important feature of the empathic response is that the
professional must identify the patient's emotion – not necessarily
experience it personally. (If the professional does experience the
same emotion as the patient, those feelings are more accurately
termed, in clinical terminology, "sympathetic" rather than empathic.) Any professional is therefore capable of formulating an
empathic response for all patients, provided that the feelings that
the patient describes are understood. It is not necessary to "cry or
bleed for every patient" in order to be able to respond supportively
to a patient's distress.

However, it is always essential to identify any strong emotion
in the room. Strong emotions cannot be ignored: if they are not
acknowledged in some way they will render the rest of the interaction useless. Whether the emotion is anger, sadness, shock,

grief, or any other emotion – and whether it is the patient that is feeling it or you, the professional – if the emotion is not acknowledged between you, then further communication will be impossible. The situation is analogous to what happens in any social embarrassment, such as when your dinner guest has spinach on a tooth – until the situation is acknowledged, everyone else's attention is fixed on the cause of the awkwardness and nobody will be able to talk normally until it has ben remedied.

> **Ground Rule: Strong emotions make communication impossible if you try to ignore them. Always try to *identify* and then *acknowledge* strong feelings – whether they are the patient's or yours.**

The form of the empathic response can be as simple as restating the expressed emotion and its source.

> *Scenario 1:* A young woman has just been told she has genital herpes.
> *Patient says:* "This makes me really furious. That boyfriend of mine has certainly got some explaining to do."
> *Empathic response:* "You sound really angry at catching herpes from your boyfriend."

This response will allow the patient to elaborate and perhaps include her suspicion that her boyfriend has been unfaithful.

> *Scenario 2:* The patient is seen after a long wait in the waiting room.
> *Patient says:* "Do you realize you kept me waiting for nearly two hours in that waiting room?!"
> *Empathic response:* "It must be extremely frustrating to be kept waiting for such a long time."

This response may precipitate elaboration of the anger (*Of course it's frustrating ...*), but the anger has been acknowledged. To avoid all mention of it will cause increasing tension and will probably halt meaningful communication between you and the patient.

   Part of your ability to interpret patients' feelings will depend on your knowledge of their social and family circumstances. This is the point at which the "social history" is of real help in aiding your understanding of some of a person's reactions. I do not mean to imply that you have to learn everything about all the social circumstances of every single patient; but if you are having difficulty in assessing the impact of an illness on a patient, one way of approaching it is to find out more about the patient's social environment. As a simple example: a loss of two months' wages after a fracture might be survivable for a comfortable professional family, but might spell disaster for a family surviving near the poverty level.

Silence: Not all silences are the same. Some silences or pauses, when the patient is struggling to find the words, facilitate the interview. Other silences, particularly when emotions are running high, serve a more important function. Your silence can give the patient permission to feel, express, or display emotions. Such a silence on your part at that point can be a deliberate response, not merely a facilitation technique. There are occasions in which this silence (accompanied by touch if appropriate) can be an important part of your dialogue – when there seems to be nothing to say because there is nothing to say. None of us needs to be particularly afraid of the spaces between words.

These, then, are the major categories of response. We shall now look at various ways in which you might use them.

Open questions vs empathic responses

The empathic response, because it depends on your interpretation of the patient's emotions, is an intuitive leap. In other words, the professional is guessing what the patient is feeling. If you are correct, you will have speeded up the interview, and brought yourself closer to your patient's view of the situation in a short time. If you are wrong, you may create some problems. As an example:

> *Patient:* "... and my period's late, so I think I'm pregnant."
> *Doctor:* "You must be delighted."

Here, if the doctor happens to be wrong (by misjudging the patient's expressions or appearance), the patient may react angrily, or may be distressed or depressed. In any event, the patient will trust the doctor less.

The best guideline is a simple one: if you are fairly sure that you know what the patient is feeling, use an empathic response. If you are not sure, use an open question. In the above example, an appropriate open question might be something like this:

Patient: "... and my period's late, so I think I'm pregnant."
Doctor: "How would you feel if you were?"

This can be rephrased as a

> **Ground Rule: Empathic responses are shortcuts. Use them if you are sure where you are going. If you are not sure, use open questions** *until you are clear about what the patient is feeling and why.*

One further point about empathic responses and open questions. Both of these devices bring you closer to the patient's view of the situation – both are, as it were, range finders. But they only work it you listen intently to the patient's response. The efficiency with which they bring you close to the patient-depends on your concentration.

Finally, a word of encouragement: certainly, these techniques (open questions and empathic responses) are more tiring than any automatic answer or a brush-off. However, those "easier" responses (especially hostile responses) will only buy you (at best) a short time of tranquillity. We all may feel better having shouted at a patient, but we will have to face him or her (or a lawyer!) at the next interview, so that any peace is likely to be short-lived. These responses involve harder work, but the yields are higher and the relationship gets easier with time.

> **Ground Rule: Both the open question and the empathic response place considerable demands on your energy. Using an open question requires more effort as you listen to the patient's response; the empathic response requires your concentration as you frame it.**

Open questions vs closed questions

As we have already seen, the closed question is the staple of the history-taking interview and is something which all professionals are familiar. There is nothing intrinsically wrong with using closed questions for other parts of the medical interview (even when the subject matter is breaking bad news). In practice, however, there is a temptation to use closed questions as a means of avoiding contentious issues. Then the closed question causes problems. Here is an example of a closed question being used to avoid dealing with a patient's distress:

> Scenario: A young woman has just come to her family practi-
> tioner with a complaint of loss of appetite and insomnia. Her
> mother has recently been diagnosed as having a recurrence of
> her previously treated bladder cancer.
> Patient: "... and when my mother said the doctor told her
> the cancer had come back I was so upset I could hardly
> breathe."
> Doctor: "Did you get any chest pain with that shortness of
> breath?"

If there were genuine reasons to expect that the patient might have a cardiac problem (for instance, if the doctor were meeting an older patient for the first time who presented with symptoms of decreased exercise tolerance), the question might be legitimate. In the scenario illustrated here, however, the question is clearly an attempt by the doctor to avoid dealing with the main feature of the patient's statement: *I was so upset.*

In most of the examples that follow later in chapter 5, we shall be seeing ways in which closed questions can be misused to avoid ussues. Occasionally, however, we shall see that a closed question can be used appropriately to further define a patient's emotional state. Here is an example:

> Scenario: As above.
> Patient: "... and when my mother said the doctor told her
> the cancer had come back I was so upset I could hardly
> breathe."
> Doctor: "Was it the thought that your mother might die that
> made you so upset?"

Be aware, therefore, that in later chapters we will usually be using closed questions as examples of camouflage for a retreat. However, some examples will show how a closed question can be used appropriately to help define the emotional content of a situation more precisely.

If closed questions are usually best avoided when the emotional temperature is rising, there is no reason why you should avoid open questions. One of the most common – and perhaps one of the most important – pitfalls in any medical interview is when the professional doesn't know exactly what the patient is feeling, and is aware of that ignorance, but feels that he or she ought to know. This usually causes a sense of embarrassment in the professional. If you find yourself in this position, try to use an open question to find out more of what is going on, instead of continuing and getting into deeper waters.

Here is a simple example in which the patient's statement doesn't tell the doctor what the patient is really concerned about. The open question used here allows the patient to air the issue:

> *Patient:* "... then my mother died and I thought I should get a checkup."
> *Doctor:* "What were you thinking about in particular?"

Obviously there are many different things that the patient might be worried about. Bland reassurance from the physician, or even something like *Right, let's check you over*, will avoid airing the major concerns, whereas an open question invites the patient to air the biggest worries.

Different responses to a patient's anger

Now we can look at several different responses and compare their impact on the interview. In the example on p. 62 (and in the many that follow the same pattern, particularly in chapter 5) we will see the many crossroads in doctor-patient interviews. Initially, a clinical interview might seem to be linear, moving from start to finish in a way that depends mainly on the personality or mood of the patient. In reality, the interview is much more flexible than one might suppose and the direction of the interview can be changed at many points. Each of the types of response mentioned above will have a different impact on the interview, and the objective of the following diagram is to demonstrate the directions in which the interview will probably move after each type. These responses are not the only ones – nor are they the ones you would necessarily

Scenario: A patient has newly diagnosed AIDS presenting with pneumocystis pneumonia.

Patient says: *I've got AIDS and you're no damned use. You can't cure it.*

You might respond:

CLOSED QUESTION
How quickly did you go to your own doctor after the cough started? (1)

HOSTILE RESPONSE
Look, no one can cure AIDS – that's something you should have thought about sooner. (2)

OPEN QUESTION
How does that make you feel? (3)

EMPATHIC RESPONSE
It must make you very angry to have this disease and not be able to control it. (4)

(1)   This is almost a biased question (being a defensive response), blaming the patient for any delay. It may negate any later attempts to be of support to the patient.

(2)   This will cause escalation into a full-scale argument and breakdown in the relationship.

(3)   This may well be followed by an outburst of anger: however, you will be in the position of someone who is available to listen, and as the outburst subsides, you will clearly be seen in the role of a support to the patient.

(4)   This identifies the reaction and the cause of it and attempts to articulate both. Having acknowledged the patient's anger you can continue (... *and who wouldn't feel angry, but let's talk about what can be done to help* ...) and stay on track as the clinician in charge of the patient instead of being isolated by the patient's anger.

choose. They simply illustrate a few of the responses that might occur to some or all of us in the given settings.

In the example on p. 62, we have set out four of the many responses that you might make when confronted by a patient expressing anger. Depending on your own personality, inclinations, manners, and mood you might previously have thought of only one of these, and regarded that one exclusively as the "right and proper" way to respond.

Professional vs social dialogue

Finally, we need to comment briefly on the differences between social conversations and professional conversations (that is, interviews). There is no doubt that professional interviews are facilitated by some social interactions, and that putting a patient at her or his ease is an important part of a successful interview. However, the professional relationship (and therefore the professional interview) contains an implicit contract between the health care professional and the patient that is absent from social interactions.

The contract is based on the fact that the professional person (doctor, nurse, student, or other staff member) has access to professional knowledge and expertise that puts her or him at an advantage over the patient. The codes of all medical professions are based on the understanding that the professional partner will not use that knowledge to the disadvantage of the patient or client. In other words, the potential vulnerability of the patient is protected by the code of professional behaviour incumbent on the professional person. This has major implications for the nature of the interview. During all the discussions that follow, it is always understood that the professional person is obliged to use her or his professional abilities for the benefit of the patient (the concept in medical ethics of "beneficence"). This obligation limits the number of permissible options available to you. And rightly so – none of us, as a professional, is permitted to say or do simply anything that we wish: being professional means that we have to honour certain obligations to our patients.

SUMMARY

1   Preparing to listen:
     – sit down, look relaxed

2   Questioning:
     – closed questions for the history
     – open questions for the rest

3   Effective listening (facilitating):
     – start the patient talking
     – encourage continuation

4   Hearing:
     – repetition, reiteration

5   Responding:
     – responses can be questions or statements
     – appropriate responses include: open and closed ques-
       tions, factual or empathic responses (identifying the
       emotion and its cause and acknowledging them), and
       silence
     – responses do not have to be the complete answer

FURTHER READING

Bernstein L, Bernstein RS. Interviewing: a guide for health professionals.
   Norwalk, CT: Appleton Century Crofts, 1985
Billings JA, Stoeckle JD. The clinical encounter. Chicago: Year Book Medical
   Publishers, 1989
Cassell E. Talking with patients. 2 vols. Cambridge, MA: Massachusetts
   Institute of Technology, 1985
Hall ET. The silent language. New York: Doubleday, 1959
Ley P. Communicating with patients. London: Croom Helm, 1988
Roter D, Stewart M, eds. Communication with medical patients. Newbury
   Park: Sage Publications, 1989

4 Breaking Bad News: A Six-Step Protocol

Some general comments

THE NATURE OF A "BREAKING BAD NEWS" INTERVIEW

The interview in which bad news is discussed is an asymmetric one: you have information to impart that the patient does not (yet) possess. However, the patient's responses are in some respects the most crucial part of the interview. You can think, therefore, of the interview as having two components:

- a divulging of information: by which you impart information to the patient
- a therapeutic dialogue: by which you listen to, hear, and respond to the patient's reactions to the information

The division is, of course, spurious since both transactions go on simultaneously, but for the sake of clarity, we will consider the two components separately. In this chapter we will set out the structure or protocol for the divulging of information, and in chapter 5 we will present an analysis of the patient's possible reactions and feelings, and the subsequent options available to the professional.

Once again, it should be stressed that the protocol outlined in this chapter is only a guideline. However, it seems to be in accord with much research work in the field, and in particular it matches the perspective-display series as described by Maynard.[46]

Most of us, as professionals, are at our worst when we have no plan at all, and a set of guidelines enhances competence and decreases feelings of unease for all concerned. What follows here is not therefore a rigid agenda to which you must inflexibly adhere; it is a track through what appears to be, at first, an untrackable area. With experience, we all find other tracks and devise our own routes.

HOW MUCH TIME DOES THIS NEED?

This protocol is intended for use in busy clinical practice. You can use these techniques in an average general practice, if you are a physician or a nurse on a busy medical ward, or anywhere else. The luxury of having two hours of contemplation with each patient is not required. (In fact, there is good evidence to show that a patient's satisfaction does not depend on the amount of time spent.[47]) With increasing experience, we all learn which are the most important topics to deal with, and in what circumstances it is safe to cut corners. The process is similar to learning the elements of the physical examination – it is necessary for medical students to learn the examination of every body system because physical signs in one might be crucial in an individual case. After a time, however, physicians learn to abbreviate the examination of, say, the peripheral sensory system in a patient awaiting an elective hernia repair. The same is true of breaking bad news: as time goes on, interviewing skills become more efficient, getting to the patient's major concerns more quickly and spending more time where it is most needed.

ADVOCACY

Whoever takes the main responsibility for breaking bad news to the patient, all other health care professionals involved in the patient's care may contribute to the support after the patient has heard the news. Support of the patient involves time spent listening, hearing, and acknowledging the emotions that the patient is experiencing, and also advocacy on the patient's behalf. The word advocacy literally means "speaking for" the patient. Whatever your relationship with the patient and whatever your role on the health care team, it is always possible to assist the patient in framing his or her main fears and anxieties, and to help him or her obtain information about the questions you cannot answer from other staff who may have the information.

In order to do this, it is necessary to accept that there are questions that you personally cannot answer. Accept them as problems central to the patient's view of the situation, and take them to a potential source of answers. This act of advocacy is an extremely valuable service for the patient.

In fact, non-physician staff (particularly medical students and junior nurses) are quite often specifically targeted by patients for the most difficult questions, because they are clearly members of the team but appear to be non-threatening and may still be "on the patient's side." Furthermore, the fact that a junior team-member might not know the answers is another attractive feature if the patient is ambivalent and uncertain whether she or he really wants to hear the medical facts.

> **Ground Rule: If you can't answer a question, don't try.**
> **Instead, it is always possible to act as the patient's advocate**
> **– listen to the question and take it elsewhere for further**
> **information.**

The Six-Step Protocol

The six basic steps of the protocol will now be described individually. In the appendix of the book, you will find a transcript of an interview with a (simulated) patient with newly diagnosed acute leukemia that shows how the six steps fit together in continuous conversation.

STEP 1. GETTING STARTED

Getting the physical context right
Starting off is always difficult, but, as the proverb goes, even the longest journeys begin with a single step. It is also true, however, that the first step is one of the most crucial, since it is more difficult and time-consuming to correct the course later if you have moved in the wrong direction initially.

Unless it is absolutely unavoidable, an interview about bad news should be carried out in person and not over the telephone. A recent study[48] showed that when doctors disclosed bad news over the telephone they were perceived as being less helpful by the patients. Occasionally there is no alternative, and you have to make do with a telephone conversation (there are some suggestions about this approach in chapter 6); but if it is humanly possible, this is part of the doctor-patient interaction that should always be person-to-person.

In practical terms, whenever you start an interview about bad news, spend a few seconds getting the physical context right – or as right as possible (as detailed in chapter 3).

> **Ground Rule: Always try to get the physical setting right: if you do so you will, first, reassure yourself (because you are in control, and doing something with which you are familiar) and, second, reassure your patient (because you look more relaxed, and seem to know what you are doing).**

Where?
If possible, take the patient and/or relative to a separate room so you can all sit down in privacy. It has to be said that in most clinical settings this isn't possible, but even when an interview room is available, most doctors don't use it because they are uncomfortable with "the long walk."

> **Practice Point:** You can always cover "the long walk" with an explanation such as *I know it's a bit of a walk, but it'll be much easier to talk if we can sit down* or *You'll find it easier to ask questions if we find somewhere quiet and private.* Again, in doing

this, you are taking command of the situation, which makes for less discomfort all round.

If there is no interview room available and the patient is an in-patient, draw the curtains (which gives an illusion of privacy and makes neighboring patients or visitors aware that they shouldn't be listening, although they certainly will be). If you are in the patient's home, close the door (which seems obvious, but is often forgotten, causing the patient to feel even more vulnerable).

Very rarely you may have to conduct interviews standing up (if there is absolutely nowhere to go and the interview has to be held that moment). In that case, take the person (most likely a relative) aside and stand a little closer than you would normally, minimizing the chances of being separated by passersby pushing through. However ludicrous it may sound, crucial conversations in corridors are quite commonly interrupted by orderlies pushing food-trolleys between a doctor and relative.

> **Practice Point:** If it is unavoidable that the interview has to be carried out standing up, leaning against the wall at least gives an illusion that the professional is there to stay for some time and not about to run away. It is not optimal, but it's better than nothing.

Who should be there?
If there is a visitor with the patient, ask her or him – gently – who they are or what relationship they have to the patient (*Are you a relative of Mrs. Brown?*).

> **Practice Point:** Guessing is hazardous. On a few occasions you might find yourself asking the husband if he is the father of the patient, or the wife if she is the mother. It is difficult to dig your way out of something like that. One of our colleagues once had an extremely important conversation in front of someone whom he thought was the father of the patient but who was actually a visiting priest who knew the patient only slightly (*This is Father Charles ...*). It was not a disaster, but it easily could have been.

If there is another person there, and neither the patient nor the
visitor shows any inclination to end the visit, ask the patient if he
or she would like to continue the interview with the visitor present.
(If the visitor is the spouse, you may say something like ... *and I
assume you're happy to have me talk about your condition with your
husband present*, which at least gives the patient a chance of privacy
however awkward requesting it may be (see also chapter 6).

Begin using your facilitating and effective-listening techniques
straightaway (see chapter 3), even before you have started on your
agenda, to ensure that you are attentive to what the patient is
saying or indicating.

Starting off

Attend to the normal courtesies, making sure the patient is covered
up, using the appropriate name, keeping a comfortable distance,
and paying some attention to your own body language. Then,
unless the patient begins with a question, it is a good idea to start
the conversation with some form of question (*How are you feeling
at the moment?* or *How are things today?* or even *Do you feel well
enough to talk for a bit?*). It is important to know if the patient is
in a bad state before launching into a sensitive conversation, since
it is clearly inadvisable to attempt a meaningful conversation if
the patient is nauseated or in pain or has just had a sedative drug.
Sometimes the need for the interview is pressing and you simply
may have to proceed (for instance, *I know you're not feeling well,
but perhaps we could talk for a few minutes now, then I could come
back tomorrow*).

Starting the interview in this way sends several important messages to the patient: (1) it gives the patient the idea that you are
interested in his or her condition; (2) it demonstrates that the conversation is going to be two-way; (3) it gets the patient talking;
and (4) it allows you to assess something of the patient's current
medical symptoms, mental state, and vocabulary – all of which
may be important if you do not happen to know the patient very
well.

STEP 2. FINDING OUT HOW MUCH THE PATIENT KNOWS

The next step is to obtain from the patient an impression of what he or she already knows about the illness – in particular, how serious he or she thinks it is, and how much it will affect the future. This is a crucial component of the interview, requiring full concentration and maximum listening skills, and there are many ways in which this information can be obtained. In all cases, the objective is to establish what the patient knows about the impact of the illness on his or her future, not about the basic pathology or nomenclature of her or his diagnosis. Here are some of the phrases that can be used:

> *What have you made of the illness so far?*
>
> *What have you been thinking about this nausea/ unsteadiness/breast lump/ ... ?*
>
> *Have you been very worried about this illness/these symptoms?*
>
> *What did the previous doctors tell you about the illness/ operation?*
>
> *Have you been thinking that this illness might be serious?*
>
> *Have you been worried about yourself?*
>
> *When you first had the Symptom X, what did you think it might be?*
>
> *What did Doctor X tell you when he sent you here?*
>
> *Did you think something serious was going on when ... ?*

As the patient replies, listen to the response in detail. The reply will give important information on three major aspects of the patient's situation:

1. The patient's understanding of the medical situation
How much has she or he understood, and how close to the medical reality is that impression? Some patients may, at this point, say

that they have been told nothing at all. This may or may not be true, but even if you know it to be false, accept the patient's statement as a symptom of denial and do not confront it immediately. First, the patient may be about the request information from you, and may semideliberately deny previous information to see if you tell the same story (another reason for sticking as closely to the truth as possible). Second, if the patient has been given information and is now in denial, you are unlikely to appear to be supportive if you launch an immediate confrontation.

> **Practice Point:** A patient denying previous information quite often precipitates anger or resentment on the professional's part (*My goodness, doesn't Dr. Smythe tell his patients what he found at the operation?!*). If you find yourself feeling this, beware! You may be seeing a patient in denial and you may be suffering from the syndrome we term the "nobody-ever-tells-their-patients-anything-until-I-do" syndrome. It commonly occurs when patients are sick and the emotional atmosphere is highly charged.

2. The style of the patient's statements
You may pay particular attention to the patient's emotional state, educational level, and abilities in articulation by the manner in which she or he is speaking. Listen to the vocabulary: what kinds of words is the patient using, and what kinds of words is the patient avoiding? As will be seen in step 4, it is important to determine the patient's level of understanding and articulation so that the professional can later begin the information-giving at the same level.

If the patient says *My family doctor thought it might be multiple sclerosis and I'm told the visual-evoked potentials show optic neuritis*, then clearly a lot of ground has already been covered. If the patient says *The surgeon said the breast lump was a lesion and I was so glad it wasn't a tumor or even worse, a cancer*, then (equally clearly) the information-giving will have to start at the beginning.

> **Practice Point:** Take *no* notice of the patient's profession in making this assessment. This is particularly true if your patient

is a member of a health care profession – for instance, another doctor or nurse. Far too often you will find yourself making assumptions. Even physicians when they are patients may not be experts in their own disease, and may not understand something like *It's only a Stage II but I don't like the mitotic index* when they are hearing it as a patient. It is even more important to follow these guidelines when the patient is a professional (and you may wish to cover this with something like *I know you're a nurse/doctor, but I hope you won't mind if I treat you as a human being. We'll start at the beginning and if I'm covering old ground you tell me*).

3. The emotional content of the patient's statements
There are two major sources here, verbal and nonverbal:
- *verbal:* Try to assess the emotions that the patient is talking about, and the emotions that the words imply. Also try to obtain a clear picture of what emotions the patient is trying *not* to talk about (see chapter 5).
- *nonverbal:* What other clues are being given (sitting back away from the doctor, hunched forward, crying, tight hand-wringing, and so on)? It is important to look for discordance between verbal and nonverbal communication. For example, if the hands are showing anxiety and the words are spoken with calm bravery, take note: major anxiety exists and is being suppressed.

Note that you are not required to judge these responses. You do not have to (and usually cannot) decide whether they are normal or abnormal. They are simply clues as to the patient's emotional state, and this is the moment for first trying to inform yourself about them.

To summarize the interview so far: you have minimized discomfort (the patient's and yours) as far as is possible, and the patient knows that you are trying to listen and that you are interested in what she or he thinks is going on. The next stage is pivotal in determining the further course of the interview and, to a certain extent, the future course of your relationship with the patient.

STEP 3. FINDING OUT HOW MUCH THE PATIENT WANTS TO KNOW

If there is such a thing as a critical step or choice in an interview, it is this one – the point at which it is established overtly whether or not the patient wishes to know what is going on. Even though this step is critical, as step 2 is, it is not necessarily difficult in itself. The process can be compared to a surgical incision that is clearly essential to the operation and has to be appropriately located, although in itself it is not the most difficult part of the surgery. In the same way, this component of the bad-news interview is crucial but not particularly difficult. Omitting this stage, however, leaves the subsequent parts of the interview on very delicate and insecure grounds (unless the patient has previously made a strong statement about wanting or not wanting information). Without a clear invitation (or declination) from the patient to share information, you will feel unsure of whether you are giving the patient too much or too little information.

Many of the students that we teach in Toronto express initial reservations about asking patients directly what they want to know. They think that it is "giving the game away" and that in making this inquiry you are telling the patient that she or he does have something serious, and therefore that you are not "playing fair." These reservations arise from two assumptions: first, that the question is a false one, since by the act of asking the question you are removing from the patient one of the choices that you seem to be offering (that is, the option of not discussing the situation); and second, that asking the patient's views will cause distress that might be avoidable. Both of these difficulties arise from a misunderstanding of the function of the patient's denial.

In any conversation about bad news, the real issue is not *Do you want to know?* but *At what **level** do you want to know what's going on?* Despite common illusions to the contrary, doctors' statements are not the only source of information available to patients. Patients know how they feel, they know that they are being sent for tests or for surgery, they know what other patients say, what other staff members say, and if the doctors say nothing they know that they are not hearing good news about a simple reassuring diagnosis. If the patient is using denial he or she is able to insulate himself or herself against the impact of all this – and will do the same against the impact of the question *What do you want to know?* In other words, at some level every patient knows (or will know) when things are not going well: in asking the patient about information-sharing, you are simply finding out whether or not the patient wants the information discussed overtly and in full view or not.

Several studies and detailed case histories[49] confirm that more distress is caused by not discussing the information than by discussing it. In one study[50] a physician told two hundred patients with lung cancer that the diagnosis would be available at the next visit – if they wished to know, they should ask, but if they did not wish to know they should not ask, and they would not be told. Almost exactly 50 percent of the patients asked to be told the diagnosis at the next visit, and of the other 50 percent (who did not ask to be told) half later indicated that they wished they had not been told. These results are extremely important. First, they show that you cannot make any assumptions about who wants to know and, second, you have a very low chance of doing any harm in asking. (It should be noted that several subsequent studies have found that the proportion of patients who want to know is higher than 50 percent and is in the range of 75–97 percent – see chapter 1.)

Therefore, asking the patients what they want allows them to exercise their preferences; the majority will wish for full disclosure. Those who do not, however, will not be robbed of their chance of using their denial mechanisms, and additional distress is not a common sequela.

Phrasing the question: The actual way in which you phrase the question is largely a matter of your own style, but here are some examples:

> *If this condition turns out to be something serious, are you the kind of person who likes to know exactly what's going on?*

> *Would you like me to tell you the full details of the diagnosis?*

*Are you the kind of person who likes the full details of
what's wrong – or would you prefer just to hear about the
treatment plan?*

*Do you like to know exactly what's going on or would you
prefer me to give you the outline only?*

*If your condition is serious, how much would you like to
know about it?*

*Would you like me to tell you the full details of your condition
– or is there somebody else that you'd like me to talk to?*

With all of these approaches, if the patient does not want to hear
about the full details you have not cut off all lines of communication. You are saying overtly that you will maintain contact and
communication (for example, concerning the treatment plan),
though not about the details of the disease. A phrase such as *the
sort of person who* may be particularly valuable because it suggests
to the patient that there are many patients like this, and that if he
or she prefers not to discuss the information, this is not unique,
and he or she is not suffering from extraordinary feebleness or
lack of courage.

The objective of this part of the interview should be to get a
clear invitation (if that is what the patient wishes) to share information. If the patient expresses a preference not to discuss the
information, you should leave the door open for later (for instance,
*That's fine. If you change your mind or want any questions answered
at future visits, just ask me at any time. And I won't push information
at you if you don't want it*).

Case History: Ms. Hampton was in her late sixties when she
was first seen, presenting with hepatomegaly and ascites. An
ultrasound showed that she had multiple hepatic metastases,
and that the primary was probably pancreatic. She was bedrid-
den. When asked how much she wanted to know, she replied
*If it's something bad, don't tell me about it. I haven't got any fam-
ily and I'll trust you to look after me.* She was clearly not distressed by her lack of mobility and abdominal distension, and
communicated normally and easily with everyone including a

longtime friend of hers who visited frequently. Pain control
was excellent and she remained completely calm until her
death three weeks later.

First reactions: One's first reaction in seeing a patient who is
only three weeks away from death and who doesn't want to
talk about it might have been *How can this woman ignore her
circumstances?*

Second thoughts: On reflection, it seemed that the denial and
ignoring were at an overt level only. This patient was aware of
her state but did not want it discussed it overtly. Had she
shown marked signs of fear or distress (see below) or had
there been some medical reason for major intervention, the
medical team might have pressed on further, as will be discussed in the next scenario. However, in this case, the patient
was plainly indicating that she was at ease and did not wish to
talk about the diagnosis.

In this case, there was no treatment that would have radically
altered the prognosis (despite overly optimistic claims in the medical literature). If, however, there is a treatment modality that would
make a significant difference, the patient should have (and has a
right to) full information in order to reach an informed decision
about treatment. The following case illustrates that situation. The
patient here had Stage III carcinoma of the ovary in which plat-
inum-based chemotherapy has a 50–60 percent response rate and
offers a median survival period of approximately eighteen months,
with a small percentage of patients surviving several years.

> **Case History:** Mrs. Geraldson was a senior personnel officer in
> a large corporation. The letter from the referring doctor said
> *She will simply not allow me to tell her what is going on, and I
> am concerned that you may not be able to offer her treatment.* She
> was an exceptionally nervous woman (in fact, she was so nerv-
> ous that she sat with the chair tipped back against the wall,
> with her body leaning as far back as possible and her head
> against the wall). Here first words as the physician entered the
> room were *If it's cancer, I don't want you to tell me.* The physi-
> cian assured her that he would not and asked about her fears
> of cancer. She replied that five members of her family died

many years ago of cancer and that their suffering had been extreme. Her main fears now were of similar suffering, and she
believed that if she knew it was cancer, all the fight would go
out of her. After the medical history and examination, the physician then described the treatment and its side effects in detail
and mentioned the various support services that could be offered. When she heard about the treatment, she recognized it
as chemotherapy. When the physician confirmed this and said
that he would recommend chemotherapy for her, she smiled
broadly (for the first time) and said *Oh well, I knew it was cancer anyway.* From that moment on, she relaxed and was able to
tolerate the treatments and all subsequent events with considerable calm.

The central point of this case history is that Mrs. Geraldson overtly
wished to use denial but was clearly in deep distress. Second, she
needed to have some information about her condition in order to
make an informed decision about treatment (though it would still
have been possible to give her chemotherapy with her consent
even if she had persisted in her desire not to hear the name of
her disease, provided that she understood the nature of the treatment and its complications).

This view of denial is somewhat controversial – some authorities
believe that all denial is intrinsically wrong and obstructive to the
patient's progress. As is evident, the present authors do not share
that view. Some patients need denial to acclimatize themselves to
their condition; others use it as a buffer against distress. Provided
that it is helping the patient adapt to his or her circumstances (as
it did with Ms. Hampton, but not with Mrs. Geraldson), and it is
not preventing adaptation or adding to distress, then there seems
to be no benefit to the patient in confronting it.

So far, then, we have seen how to start off the interview and
how to find out how much the patient knows and wants to know.
In the next section we shall deal with the general rules about
information-sharing. The rest of the book then focuses on this part
of the interview and what transactions can occur between professional and patient during information-sharing.

STEP 4. SHARING THE INFORMATION (ALIGNING AND EDUCATING)

Thus far, if the patient has indicated that he or she wants to know everything about the illness, we know that as we proceed we are doing so by invitation. If the patient has said that he or she does not want to know the details of the illness, we can discuss the treatment plan and the way in which the patient will be looked after (see the previous section). No matter how awkward or embarrassing it may seem to ask patients what they wish to know, the explicit agreement that emerges makes the rest of the interview far more comfortable than it would otherwise have been.

We should now consider the general rules for the transaction known as information-sharing. As we stated earlier, the interview in which bad news is discussed is an asymmetric one: you have information to impart that the patient does not (yet) possess. However, the patient's responses are in some respects the most crucial part of the interview. As we have already seen, the interview has two components:

- the divulging of information: by which the professional imparts information to the patient
- therapeutic dialogue: by which the professional listens to, hears, and responds to the patient's reactions to the information

As we stated at the start of this chapter, this division is somewhat spurious since both transactions go on simultaneously, but for the sake of clarity we will consider the two components separately (setting out an analysis of the dialogue or interchange component – the patient's possible reactions and feelings, and your subsequent options – in chapter 5).

Decide on your objectives (Diagnosis / Treatment Plan / Prognosis / Support)

Even before you start this part of the interview, you should have some idea of what you are trying to achieve with the interview. Obviously this depends partly on the patient's disease-status and partly on your own role in the health care team in relation to the patient. (If you are not the physician in charge of the patient, it may not be in your brief to explain the treatment plan, although you can still act as an advocate for the patient – as discussed at the opening of this chapter – and find out how much the patient understands, and what his or her main concerns are.)

In any event, it is essential to have some form of agenda in mind: without it, the interview is very likely to get bogged down and leave both you and the patient feeling confused.

The four crucial objectives for structuring your agenda are:

1 Diagnosis,
2 Treatment plan,
3 Prognosis, and
4 Support.

Obviously the amount of information to be shared on each of these points depends on the disease, the treatment options, the patient's preferences and reactions, and so on. We shall be dealing with some of these aspects as they crop up in the examples in chapters 5 and 6, but it seems obvious that the details of the information are those of the practice of medicine itself, and are beyond the scope of this book (or any other). No book can tell you what to say, but the authors hope that this book will help you work out how to say it.

It is often easiest to state the rough outline of the interview before beginning this part (perhaps with a comment such as *I'll start off telling you about the disease and the treatment, then we can discuss all of that and the future and anything else*). Whether or not you state your own agenda overtly at the beginning of the interview depends on you and on your patient's expectations. You do not have to have everything neatly mapped out in you mind (that is often difficult or even impossible), but you do have to have some idea of what you want to achieve during the interview.

> **Ground Rule: It is not essential to state your own agenda:
> but it is essential to have one (or at least part of one).**

Your goals may not be the same as the patient's and we shall see at the end of this section how you may try to blend the two. However, from the beginning you have to accept two inviolable rights of the patient: a mentally competent and informed patient has the right (1) to accept or reject any treatment offered and (2) to react to the news and express her or his own feelings in any (legal) way she or he chooses. These two points may seem obvious, but many interviews end in frustration because the professional feels that the patient has to accept the proffered treatment or has to react to the news just received in a certain way.

> Ground Rule: The competent and informed patient has the right to accept or reject any of your suggestions and to express any emotions in any way (within the law!).

Start from the patient's starting point (Aligning)

At this point in the interview, therefore, you have already heard how much the patient knows about the situation, and the vocabulary in which the patient expresses it. It is essential to use this as your starting point for information-giving. Reinforce those parts of what the patient has said that are correct (using the patient's words if possible) and continue from there. It gives the patient a great deal of confidence in himself or herself (as well as in you) to realize that his or her view of the situation has been heard and is being taken seriously (even if it is being modified or corrected).

This process has been called "aligning,"[51] a useful term to describe the process by which you line up the information you wish to import on the patient's knowledge baseline.

Educating

In the next phase of the interview, having started from the patient's starting point (that is, having aligned your information with the patient's original position), you now have to bring the patient's perception of the situation closer to the medical facts as you know them.

There is no word in current usage that completely describes the transaction by which the professional brings the patient's understanding of the medical situation closer to the facts, but the word that fits best is "educating." This process may be compared, perhaps, to steering an oil tanker. It is not possible to make sudden and large course corrections or to produce quick and total responses. In fact – to pursue the oil-tanker analogy a little further

– large and acute changes may be not only counterproductive but actually dangerous, and may capsize the vessel. What is required in the educating part of the breaking-bad-news interview is the application of slow and steady guidance over the direction of the interview.

To do this, it is first necessary to assess the magnitude of the divergence between what the patient understands and the medical facts (this is the "required course correction"). Then the process of education begins, changing the patient's understanding in small steps and observing the patient's responses continuously. In this process, you should reinforce those responses from the patient that are bringing him or her closer to the facts, and emphasize the relevant medical information if it becomes apparent that the patient is moving away from an accurate understanding. The key ingredients of this component of the interview are, therefore, steady observation and continued gentle guidance of the interview's direction rather than sudden lurches. The following are the major guidelines for education.

Give information in small chunks – The warning shot: Medical information is hard for patients to digest. Studies have shown that most patients fail to retain up to 50 percent of the information given, even if it is about something simple such as an IVP. When the diagnosis is serious, the information dropout may be more substantial (*The moment you said "cancer," doctor, ... I couldn't remember a single thing from then on ...*). It is important to be continuously aware of this fact, and not to expect the patient to recall everything you have said. You, after all, may have said it on many previous occasions, but the patient is hearing it for the first time.

The cardinal rule, therefore, is to give the information in small chunks. One useful technique for starting this process is the "the warning shot." If there is apparently a large gap between the patient's expectations and the reality of the situation, you can facilitate the patient's understanding by giving a warning that things are more serious than they appear to the patient. (*Well, the situation does appear to be more serious than that ...*) and then grading the information, gradually introducing the more serious prognostic points, and waiting for the patient to respond at each stage.[52]

(*The chest X-ray shows that there is a tumor on the lung.* [Pause.] *Does that make you think of any particular questions?*)

Following the warning shot, a narrative of events can be an extremely useful technique to help the patient understand what has been happening. A narrative can provide a logical and intelligible approach to difficult issues (*When you had those bruises, your blood test showed that you weren't making some components in the blood called platelets. They're made in the bone marrow and that's why your doctor wanted a bone marrow test to see what was wrong. It was that test that showed the problem ...*). This approach is not only easy to follow and remember but also helps the patient to frame his or her questions as the story continues.

As the explanation of the medical situation continues, it is important to pay particular attention to the vocabulary that you are using. The second major guideline is, therefore, to ...

Use English not Medspeak: The languages that health care professionals use for transmissing information are highly efficient and precise. They are capable of transferring a large amount of data about a patient from professional to professional in a short time (think, for example, of the brief histories presented on ward-rounds or in telephone calls from a resident in the emergency department to a staff physician). The languages of all health care professions – medspeak, nursespeak, psychspeak, and so on – are extremely useful, but they are only intelligible to the initiated. They are, in other words, esoteric languages; the patient does not understand them and feels excluded. Worse still, some words in medspeak sound the same as in common English but have completely different meanings (for instance, the words "complain" and "morbid" in *the patient complains of ...* and *there is considerable morbidity* ... have different meanings than in everyday English). Hence, if the objective is to give to the patient an understanding of the medical situation, it is necessary to translate from medspeak into English.

There are other attractions inherent in our own jargons. Most professionals are (justifiably) proud of their use of their own esoteric language. We have spent a long time as professionals learning our own dialect and becoming comfortable with it, and it is a comforting refuge for us in difficult situations. Using it to explain something to a patient also makes it less likely that the patient will be able to ask difficult questions. However, as much as it comforts and reassures the professional who uses it, it will also isolate and alienate the patient who finds it unfamiliar. Therefore, during a bad-news interview it is extremely important to ensure that you are using vocabulary that is intelligible to the patient. Some examples are shown here:

Medspeak	English
Blast cells	Leukemia
Demyelination	Multiple sclerosis
Abnormal growth	Tumor (then) cancer
Space-occupying lesion	Tumor (then) cancer
The prognosis is guarded	The situation is serious

It is important to remember that in this interview we should be using words for the benefit of the listener not ourselves, and must therefore translate our language into the patient's.

Check reception frequently: It is also important to check that the message we are transmitting is being received. This is a vital part of the professional's communication skills and should be done frequently during an interview. Such pauses also serve to break up the transmitted information into small intelligible sections. Many phrases can be used to break the monologue, but here are some that may be useful in this regard:

Am I making sense?

Do you follow what I'm saying?

Does this all seem sensible to you?

This must be a bit bewildering, but do you follow roughly what I'm saying?

Do you see what I mean?

These interjections serve several important functions: (1) they demonstrate that it matters to you if the patient doesn't understand what you are saying; (2) they allow the patient to speak (many patients feel so bewildered or shocked that their voices seem to seize up, and they need encouragement and prompting to speak); (3) they allow the patient to feel an element of control over the interview; and (4) they validate the patient's feelings (that is, make those feelings legitimate subjects for discussion between you).

Reinforce and clarify the information frequently: There are several ways you can reinforce what you are telling the patient.

1. Clarification: making sure you both mean the same thing
Even when the patient seems to understand the words, they may have different meanings for her or him – even in English (as opposed to medspeak) people may have widely differing understanding of words such as "cure" or "chronic." It is important to make certain, as far as is possible, that you both mean and understand the same thing. One of the best ways of checking on this is to *get the patient to repeat the general drift of what you have been saying.* Usually the patient will manage a successful reproduction of the major points, but occasionally you can be very surprised. A patient who has been sitting quietly, nodding at appropriate intervals, may have totally missed the main drift of what you have been saying, or may have a completely different understanding of a crucial word. Clarification during this part of the interview can save major misunderstandings later.

Ground Rule: Clarification is an essential part of education.

2. Repeat important points yourself
Because it is difficult for people to retain information, particularly if the news is serious (and even more so if denial is operating), you may have to repeat crucial points several times. Accept this as a fact of life when looking after seriously ill patients. It is not the patient's fault (and doctors are not much better when they are ill). It is simply one of the limitations of the human brain when facing up to serious illness. Use an empathic response when repeating information (*I know it's difficult to remember all these facts at one go ...*).

3. Use diagrams and written messages
A few simple scribbles on the back of an envelope of a scrap of
paper may serve as helpful aide-mémoire. These can be used very
easily to explain complex chemotherapy regimens or staging op-
erations, and then may be given to the patient to take away. They
may be meaningless to anyone else, but will often remind the
patient later on of the conversation. It may also be worth writing
down the diagnosis (perhaps even adding your own name) – again,
this gives the patient a feeling of control, and a feeling that the
doctor or nurse is prepared to stand by what she or he has said.

4. Use any written or recorded material available
Some physicians tape-record the interview and give the tape to
the patient. This is certainly feasible and has been shown to reinforce the interview, but some professionals find it a little too fussy.
(On the other hand, some patients have brought along tape re-
corders and asked to record the interview. This makes the atmosphere a little forced and unnatural, but is is probably politic
not to refuse such a request.) Many specialized units now use
printed pamphlets related to the common diseases seen there. It
is important to read them yourself first before handing them to a
patient. It is embarrassing to have a detailed interview with a
patient, give him or her a pamphlet, and then hear on the return
visit *You didn't mention the cystitis as a side effect of the drug, doctor.*
You do not have to be as detailed as the pamphlet but you should
give the patient a guide (*I've told you about all the important common
problems, but there are some others you can read about in the brochure.
They're quite rare. Some people like the complete list and that's why
we have the full details in the pamphlet).*

Although these techniques may take a few seconds or minutes,
they may save a lot of time in subsequent interviews. If patients
are told that it is difficult to remember this material, they may be
encouraged to try, whereas if they are left with the feeling that
they are particularly stupid they may start out feeling angry or
resentful.

Check your communication level: As the interview progresses, you should also be conscious of the level at which you are talking to the patient. There is a temptation to talk down to the patient and to patronize. You can make yourself aware of this issue by checking your messages reception frequently (see above) and listening to the language with which the patient replies. If the patient replies using a different vocabulary, then try to adapt yours to the patient's.

In an ideal world all doctors and (adult) patients would communicate as adult-to-adult. You can check that you are giving the patient this opportunity. Occasionally patients may elect for a more parental adult-child pattern of communication: you will pick this up in their responses (see chapter 3), and should accept this, at least initially, as one of the patient's coping strategies.

Listen for the patient's concerns: There is a serious danger in proceeding through a bad-news interview without listening to the patient's own worries or concerns.

> **Case History:** The following story was told by the widow of a patient, Ted Johnson. "Ted had come from the hospital and they had told him that he had a bad heart and that it was very serious. Our family doctor was young and he came round to see us before breakfast about a week later. He kept on repeating that Ted had to draw up his will, and should get on with it quickly. We kept on saying we'd done all that, but he kept on saying we'd have to hurry, things were getting worse very quickly. I found out later from another patient in the hospital that that doctor had had two conversations with Ted like that already while he was in hospital. After that breakfast session Ted just went silent and hardly spoke to me till he died. He went from being a bouncy cheerful businessman to being a silent brooding wreck. He died nearly a year ago and every time I think of him I remember that breakfast interview with the doctor and it makes me cry."

This history shows how counterproductive it is to proceed according to your own agenda, ignoring the patient's. Ted clearly knew the prognosis, he'd made his will, and he did not want to talk about it. The doctor undoubtedly thought he was doing the

right thing, and that somehow the facts had to be forced onto
Ted. The resulting catastrophe not only turned Ted into a withdrawn suspicious wreck, but also turned his wife's grief into pathological grief, depriving her of the ability to remember Ted with
pleasure.

None of us likes doing two things at once, but unfortunately
that is what is required in an interview about bad news. While
transmitting information to the patient, the professional has simultaneously to listen for the patient's reaction and try to elicit
her or his agenda or "shopping list" of concerns and anxieties.
There will be illustrations and examples of patient's reactions in
the next chapter, but here are the basic principles.

1. Try to elicit the "shopping list"
Quite often the patent's list of most important worries is not the
same as the professional's. For example, a patient may be more
concerned about the effect of a colostomy on his or her sex life
than about the long-term complications of ulcerative colitis. Patients are frequently more worried about hair loss from chemotherapy than about the potential risk of the primary disease. You
should try to listen for the patient's concerns, then identify and
acknowledge them. You do not necessarily have to deal with them
right away, but you can say that you understand what the patient
is talking about and will return to it in a moment. Do not, however,
simply ignore what you hear.

2. Listen for the buried question
Deep personal worries may not emerge easily. Sometimes the patient asks questions while you are talking (see chapter 3). These
questions ("buried questions") are often highly significant to the
patient. When the patient does this, finish you own sentence and
then ask the patient what he or she was saying. Be prepared to
follow that train of thought from the patient – it is quite likely to
be an important one.

3. Be prepared to be led
Quite often you may draw an interview to a close and then find
that the patient wants to start part of it again. This is not simply

contrary behavior on the part of the patient. It often stems from fear and insecurity, and by restarting the interview the patient is exerting some measure of control and (in her or his view) is at least picking the site of the battle. The following incident happened to one of the authors (R.B.).

> **Case History:** "The patient was a young family physician with a strong professional interest in counselling and psychotherapy. She had breast cancer with bone metastases unresponsive to chemotherapy. During her admission she had indicated clearly that she did not wish to talk about the future or about her personal feelings. She remained uncommunicative and 'closed' on all subjects except the immediate day-to-day physical issues. I made a couple of offers to listen if she did want to talk, but did not press her. On one visit I told her that I had only a little time on that particular ward-round: we finished talking and as I got to the door and put my hand out for the door-handle she said 'What about euthanasia, then?' I turned round and sat down again, and asked her to tell me what she meant. We then had a highly valuable conversation in a relatively short time. In retrospect, she must have felt that, since I had only a short time on the ward-round, she would be able to stop the conversation easily if it became too difficult for her. This must have given her the additional incentive to start the discussion."

> **Practice Point:** If an event similar to this occurs and you do not have any time available for a proper discussion, it is still advisable to sit down again, and tell the patient that this subject is clearly very important to her and that you would like to arrange another time to have a detailed talk about it.

Try to blend your agenda with the patient's: Trying to blend your agenda with the patient's is somewhat like a merger. You are changing or accommodating to adapt to the patient's view, and it is that sense of compromise that makes the patient feel (correctly) that you are interested in supporting him or her.

As you obtain the list of concerns from the patient, acknowledge the items on it and try to include them ("blend the agendas") in the topics that you cover in your conversation. You can often state the blending quite overtly (*I know you're very worried about hair loss, and I'll come to that in a moment, but can I first cover the reasons that we recommend chemotherapy in the first place?*).

STEP 5. RESPONDING TO THE PATIENT'S FEELINGS

Identify and acknowledge the patient's reaction

The success or failure of the breaking-bad-news interview ultimately depends on how the patient reacts and how you respond to those reactions and feelings. Since the subject of the patient's reactions (and your responses to them) is so large, we have decided, for convenience, to separate our discussion of the patient's feelings and reactions into a chapter of its own (chapter 5). In that chapter we set out most of the types of responses that you will encounter and show you some of the options available to you. As you will see, this is the part of the interview that requires your most sustained and continued concentration. This is also the part in which accumulated experience will produce the greatest change and improvement, as you become progressively less surprised by patients' reactions and more able to take the twists and turns of the interview in your stride.

STEP 6. PLANNING AND FOLLOW-THROUGH

Planning for the future

At this point in the interview, depending on the severity of the bad news, the patient may well feel bewildered, dispirited, and disorganized. While you are, correctly, sensitive to those emotions and are capable of empathy, you have to do more than simply reflect the patient's emotions. The patient is looking to you (since you are a professional) to make sense of any confusion and to offer plans for the future. In fact it is this ability that distinguishes the professional from the friend or well-wisher. At this point in the interview, therefore, you have to try and put together what you know of the patient's agenda, the medical scenario, and the plan of management. It is at this stage in the interview (having listened to and heard the patient) that you should offer the clinical perspective and guidance, demonstrating that you are on the patient's side. It is not possible to do this until you have heard the patient and his or her agenda, but equally this is the part of the interview that demonstrates the professional's clinical management skills. It is in this role that the patient perceives one as being a "real" doctor / nurse / other health care professional. You can think of this stage as consisting of five basic steps:

1. Demonstrate an understanding of patient's problem list
If the interview has been going according to plan, this is what you have been doing since the beginning. From the outset, you have been using those techniques we detailed in chapter 3 (effective listening) and have been telling the patient that you have been hearing what bothers the patient most.

2. Indicate you can distinguish the fixable from the unfixable
With both medical problems and psychosocial problems, some are fixable and some are not. We shall be discussing this matter further in chapter 5 in relation to the patient's responses, but showing that you know the difference is a pragmatic step without which your support will appear to be less effective. If the interview gets stuck or bogged down as the patient explores her or his problems, it is often helpful to try to enumerate the problems as a list, getting the patient to arrange them in order of priority. You can then begin to set your own agenda, stating the problems you are going to try and tackle first. This is the part of the interview that requires the widest breadth of your knowledge as a physician, nurse, or other professional, and demands the greatest concentration in arranging your own ideas and plans in logical order.

This is the first part of the process of making a contract for the future, and it is useful not to be unrealistically overoptimistic (overbidding) about the future. Such restraint now will avoid disillusion later on.

3. Make a plan or strategy and explain it
When you make a plan for the future, it is quite permissible for that plan to include many uncertainties, "don't knows," and choices (*If the dizziness doesn't get better, then we'll ...*). What you are ac-

tually doing is presenting a decision-tree or algorithm. Patients need to know that you have some plan in mind – even if it consists of little more than *we'll deal with each problem as it arises* – which, at least, implies that you will not abandon the patient. The act of making a plan and explaining it to the patient is part of what the patient sees as support. It defines the immediate future of your relationship with this particular patient and reinforces the individuality of this person and what you are going to do for her or him. To put it another way:

> Ground Rule: The management plan includes the management of the medical condition and forms part of the support of the patient.

Preparing for the worst and hoping for the best. With the contemporary emphasis on positive attitudes, you may encounter resistance and criticism as you help patients makes plans for the worst scenarios (paralysis, for example, or deterioration and death). It is most important to realize – and to state – that the human brain is functionally compartmentalized, and is quite capable of making plans for the worst while still hoping for the best. After all, most normal people draw up a will with the express intention of dividing up their assets after they have died. Drawing up a will does not (usually) cause instant death, nor does it rob the person of his or her will to live (for a recent review on psychological attitudes and cancer see note 53). We constantly make plans and then live as if those plans will not be needed; this is part of the homeostasis of our moods. In helping patients adjust to the future, it is often worth stressing this point very clearly. A useful phrase like *preparing for the worst doesn't stop us hoping for the best* allows you to reinforce the fact that this is a normal way of functioning.

4. Identify patient's coping strategies and reinforce them
There is a lot of emphasis in professional training on what we do to patients or for our patients. In acute situations, such as diabetic coma or during an appendectomy, the professionals clearly have to do all the work since the patient is unconscious. However, in facing chronic illness, the patient can and must help himself or herself, and it is counterproductive not to assess the coping strategies and assemble the support systems that are available to the

patient. At this point in the interview, then, you should begin to look at the psychological resources (and resourcefulness) available to the patient, and begin helping the patient to evaluate what he or she can do for himself or herself. This part of the process involves helping the patient identify his or her own coping strategies; we shall illustrate some of these processes in chapter 5.

5. Identify and incorporate other sources of support
Not only do we tend to forget that the patient has capabilities of her or his own, we also tend to forget that there is anyone outside the professional-patient relationship who can assist. Most people have at least one or two friends or relatives who are close in some way and can add support. For those patients who have no social supports of their own, we have to enroll whatever social services are available in the neighbourhood. The interview about bad news is an important juncture at which to start this assessment and to incorporate other sources of support in the patient's future plans.

Supporting the patient
What does "support" mean? The word is used frequently in professional and lay articles about patients. Usually the word is undefined; often it is overused. We are constantly being told that we must support our patients and (depending on our country of origin) that we must *be there for our patients*. But what precisely do those phrases mean? There can be no doubt of the intentions and the motives, but what is this behavior called supporting, and how do we do it? The real answer to those questions touches on the fundamentals of the doctor-patient relationship and includes almost every aspect of the entire practice of medicine, but there are briefer and more practical ways of attempting to define support pragmatically.

Basically "support" for the patient does not mean handing the patient a carte blanche. You do not have to – and cannot – meet every demand or agree with everything that every patient says. However, you can hear what the patient says and identify the emotions, and that action can and should be uncritical ("nonjudgmental"). What we have called effective listening is the first component of supporting the patient. There will always be areas of difference, some based on your professional knowledge, some based on your philosophical standpoint. The existence of areas of difference does not mean that you are failing to support the patient.

> **Case History:** Ms. Hodgson was a lawyer in her mid-thirties who had recurrent carcinoma of the ovary that was resistant to platinum. She had pelvic recurrence seen on CT scan and a rising CA-125 level, but was perfectly asymptomatic. She sought many different opinions and spent a great deal of time discussing options over a period of several months, during which time she remained asymptomatic and without treatment. Eventually, she decided to try high-dose (and very toxic) therapy, even though her physicians felt that this was at best premature and at worst a loss of her valuable time (as well as money). None of her medical team "supported" her view that this therapy was the best option, but all of them did support (and acknowledge) her strong desire to try anything at whatever cost, although in their view this was likely to be counterproductive in regard to her physical health. She was assured that the team would be available to her after the therapy, and she acknowledged with gratitude the fact that support was not being withdrawn from her even though she was undertaking treatment that none of the team would recommend medically.

> **Ground Rule: To support a patient you do not have to agree with the patient's point of view, but you do have to listen to it and identify what the patient is saying.**

Making a contract / Follow-through

The final part of the interview is the summary and contract for the future. The summary, which also requires a great deal of thought, should show the patient that you have been listening and that you have picked up the main concerns and issues. It is not an easy task, but you should try to give an overview of the two agendas (your and the patient's). As we shall see in chapter 5, you do not have to provide all the solutions to all the problems – present and future – at the first discussion. It is quite permissible, honest, and commendable to indicate the uncertainties of the situation. It is often helpful to give the patient an idea of the sequential decision-tree, or algorithm, by which you will make the plan (*So we'll continue the tablets for a maximum of eight weeks, and if the unsteadiness has not improved we'll repeat the tests* or *We'll redo the chest X-ray at the time of each treatment, and if there is no improvement after two courses, then we'll stop and make a new plan*).

Having summarized the main points, you should then ask the following question (or something similar to it):

Are there any (other) questions you'd like to ask me now?

Sometimes the patient has been bottling up concerns over some issue that simply has not arisen. Sometimes it's one aspect of the treatment or the disease that you have merely touched on; or it may be a major concern or source of anxiety (or even phobia) that the patient has been keeping bottled up until overt permission for discussion (implied by your question) has been given. In any event, this portion of the interview is as important as the question period after a lecture – it is the time when any burning unresolved issues can be aired.

> **Practice Point:** Many patients – for various reasons having to do with the disease, the clinical setting, perceived intimidation, and so on – cannot think of anything to ask at that moment. It is often useful to tell patients that this is not the last chance to discuss major issues, and to encourage them to jot down any other questions that occur on a piece of paper and bring them to the next meeting. In the experience of the present authors, this invitation has never led to an inundation with hundreds of written queries. Certainly there will be the occasional patient who attends with three sheets of written questions, but that usually happens at the first interview (before the invitation to write down the important questions has been given). Even with those patients, the number of questions at subsequent interviews will almost always diminish, despite this offer.

Finally, you should make a contract for the future. This can be very simply (*I'll see you at the next visit in two weeks* or *We'll try the new anti-sickness medicine and I'll see you tomorrow on the ward-*

round), but it's very important. At the conclusion of the interview patients may be left with the feeling that there is no future, and may be glad to hear that there is one. If you are not intending to see the patient again (as is more likely to happen in tertiary referral centers), then you can at least indicate the lines of communication (*I won't make a return appointment, but if anything crops up that your family doctor wants my advice on, he can call me*). Perhaps the most important function of the summary-and-contract is to show the patient that she or he has been heard and has made an impression on you. It is, perhaps, an essential component of human nature, amplified during illness, that everybody wants to be considered as special to some extent and to somebody, and everyone dreads being ignored.

> **Ground Rule: No interview is complete without a summary-and-contract.**

SUMMARY

1   Interviews about bad news consist of
       – a component of divulging information
       – a dialogue between the professional and the patient
         that may provide a therapeutic benefit for the patient

2   Bad news itself causes distress: a supportive and sensitive
       interview may minimize the eventual amount of distress.

The Six-Step Protocol

Step 1. Start off well
   – Get the physical context right
   – Where?
   – Who should be there?
   – Starting off

Step 2. Find out how much the patient knows

Step 3. Find out how much the patient wants to know

Step 4. Share the information (Aligning and Educating)
  – Decide on your agenda (diagnosis / treatment plan /
    prognosis / support)
  – Start from the patient's starting point (Aligning)
  – Educating
    Give information in small chunks
    Use English not Medspeak
    Check reception frequently
    Reinforce and clarify the information frequently
    Check your communication level (adult–adult, etc.)
    Listen for the patient's agenda
    Try to blend your agenda with the patient's

Step 5. Responding to the patient's feelings
  – Identify and acknowledge the patient's reaction

Step 6. Planning and follow-through
  – Organizing and planning
  – Making a contract and follow-through

FURTHER READING

Billings AJ. Sharing bad news. In: Outpatient management of advanced
  cancer. New York: Lippincott, 1985: 236–59
Maynard D. Notes on the delivery and reception of diagnostic news regarding
  mental disabilities. In: Helm DT, Anderson T, Meehan JA, Rawls AW, eds.
  Directions in the study of social order. New York: Irvington, 1989

5 The Patient's Reactions

General hints in responding to reactions

In the everyday practice of breaking bad news, the difference between a skilled and an unskilled physician is seen most clearly in the abilities and techniques that each uses in coping with the patient's reactions. Compared with this task, the information-divulging component is relatively simple and can be improved with a judicious choice of words and a few general rules. The difficult (and infinitely variable) component of the interview arises when patients start reacting – and this begins as you enter the room (or usually before), whether either of you realize it or not.

ASSESSMENT OF PATIENT'S RESPONSE

Trained as we are in the biomedical model of health and disease, it is very tempting to try to assess the patient's responses as either normal or pathological. There is nothing intrinsically wrong or dangerous in this process in most medical situations, but in the case of responding to patients after they have heard bad news, this approach may be inadequate and may actually serve to block communication. The range of normal reactions is very wide, and it is too easy to make a diagnosis of "abnormal reaction" in an individual case, thereafter ignoring or isolating the patient. The sensation of being cut off or ignored by medical or nursing staff as a result of an implicit judgment of behavior or response is a common and major cause of patients' dissatisfaction with the staff. This is not to imply that in responding to a patient's behavior by a patient or relative should be accepted and accommodated. However, our response to our patients' behavior does have to be more detailed and more individualized than a simple diagnosis of 'normal" versus "abnormal." In this chapter we shall set out the major guidelines and principles by which this process of individualizing can become more consistent, so that the patient is offered support that fits (or more nearly fits) that individual.

In practical terms, therefore, as professionals we require an approach by which we can assess patients' reactions and then respond to them. The most useful criteria are the following:

- *social acceptability:* a reaction has to be within the bounds of cultural norms and rules; for instance, crying is almost universally acceptable, but running amok in the clinic is not
- *adaptability:* does the reaction increase or decrease the patient's distress at his or her situation?
- *fixability:* if the reaction is increasing the patient's distress, are there any interventions that might help?

As we consider these criteria in greater detail, it is worth reinforcing the fact that the boundaries of "acceptable behavior" should be drawn up generously.

> **Ground Rule: When a patient receives bad news, the range of normal reactions is wide.**

THE PORTRAIT IN MINIATURE

Every human being develops his or her own way of dealing with misfortunes or reverses. Each of us, when confronted with bad news, will exhibit a series of reactions (some of which will help us cope with the bad news and some of which will not). When a patient hears bad news, the reaction that the professional will see is almost certainly a display of that person's accustomed method of reacting to stress – a miniature portrait or "replay" of the way that individual has handled misfortune in the past (albeit modified by advancing years, increasing maturity, and experience).

Of course, it may happen (and often does) that medical bad news is the worst thing that has befallen this person. We all tend to think of our own various financial, marital, or work-related misfortunes as the worst things that could possibly happen – until something worse actually happens. Life-threatening illness is often the worst thing that most people can imagine, and hence the reactions to it may be the most intense ever expressed by that particular person.

Thus, the mixtures of reactions unfolding in a bad-news interview are likely to be intense, and are not likely to be determined by the disease itself or by the stage of the patient's reaction (see chapter 2). They are more likely to be characteristic of that particular human dealing with a serious problem, and have evolved over the years as a result of family influences, childhood events, adult rewards, and so on. The professional's job is not to decide simply whether this mixture is normal or abnormal (compared to other people, or to some predetermined norm), but whether or not it is helping the patient cope with the situation, and, if it is not, what can be done to diminish the distress. Occasionally, a patient's behavior will be so florid and disturbing that some limits have to be set before the interview can move on to assist in resolving the issues. This is not a common occurrence, but merits some consideration.

ACCEPTABLE BEHAVIOR

A society or a culture is nothing (ultimately) but a set of rules by which a group identifies, recognizes, and contains its members. If a patient or relative behaves outside the boundaries of social acceptability, we have to say so, even though we should always err on the side of generosity in our interpretation of those boundaries. On the rare occasions when somebody does something that is simply unacceptable (smashing furniture or physically threatening a member of staff, for example), it is usually better to try to stay calm and tell him or her as firmly as you can – without getting into a rage or a panic yourself – that this behavior is not acceptable. In most instances, if the behavior does not provoke a major reaction (such as rage or fear) from you, it loses its primary gain for the patient or relative, and will resolve itself. The following instance, which happened to one of the authors (R.B.), illustrates the usefulness of avoiding a direct response to provocation.

> **Case History:** "The most aggressive behavior that I have had to face (other than from patients in the emergency department who were on drugs or going through a psychotic episode) came from a husband of a woman dying of metastatic melanoma. At the first meeting he swore continuously for several minutes about the hospital, other doctors, and me, and then started throwing a chair around the room, getting it closer and closer to me. The more he ranted, the more I tried to look calm (I stayed seated, undid my jacket, and made sure my shoulders did not hunch up, although I was quite scared) and I told him (when I could) that I would listen to whatever he had to say, but we had to talk as civilized people. When he failed to get a reaction from his violent behavior, he simply stopped and a few minutes later his behavior – although still florid – was well within the limits of acceptability."

On very rare occasions, if a calm response fails, it may be necessary to call for assistance (including security guards or police if the behavior is really threatening) as a last resort. In the great majority of cases, however, this is unnecessary and the aggressive behavior can be toned down by a firm stressing of the rules of the situation.

In some cultures, people are quite vocal and, for example, cry loudly or shriek. While this may be acceptable in the culture of the patient, it may be unacceptable, for instance, to the patient in the next bed if you are in a hospital. If it is not possible to find a room for the noisy patient or family to be noisy in, you should explain (again, as firmly and as gently as you can manage) that while you understand their strong feelings, it is essential to minimize the disturbance to other patients. Being tactful in these circumstances is not easy; however, it pays to be as firm and calm as possible.

Ground Rules for Unacceptable Behavior:
- Give as much latitude as you can.
- Try to stay calm, and speak softly.
- Be gentle while you're being firm.

DISTINGUISHING THE ADAPTIVE FROM THE MALADAPTIVE

In assessing the patient's reaction to the bad news, we now have to decide whether the response is helping the patient (and is part of the solution) or not (and is part of the problem). The process by which we make this assessment is based partly on principles that are easy to grasp and to describe, but also on clinical judgment, which is difficult to describe but which is acquired (surprisingly rapidly) as this task is performed more often.

The central principle is a simple one: some reactions may appear to the abnormal to you, but are not abnormal for that patient and may be helping the patient to recover equanimity (an adaptive response). Other reactions, by contrast, may appear to be socially or culturally desirable but may actually prevent a patient from truly coping with the news (a maladaptive response).

In complex clinical situations it may not be possible to decide instantly whether a particular response is adaptive or maladaptive. Sometimes it will require observation of the patient over a period of time to see if the distress is improving or worsening. Even though we shall try in this chapter to offer guidelines, it is important to remember that you do not have to make the diagnosis (of adaptive or maladaptive response) at first sight.

In the next section of this chapter, for most of the patient's responses we shall be highlighting those features that make them adaptive or maladaptive. For instance, as we shall discuss, denial is often viewed as an unhelpful reaction (or treated as a stage, as in the Kubler-Ross system). In our view, however, denial is part of the way in which most human beings take on board information that threatens to overwhelm them. Hence, in our way of assessing reactions, denial may be viewed as adaptive in the early stages of taking in bad news (when it may allow the patient to cope with the bad news one step at a time), but if denial is prolonged and later prevents the patient from making rational decisions, then it becomes maladaptive. It is often not possible to decide which kind it is until some time has elapsed. In the same way, some amount of crying may be part of the way a particular person copes with bad news, whereas prolonged collapse into tearfulness (say over several interviews over many days or weeks) is part of a more severe problem and is not a matter of "crying it out."

As an introduction to what we are about to deal with, here is a listing of some of the main reactions to bad news displayed by patients:

Adaptive	Maladaptive
Humor	Guilt
Denial	Pathological denial
Abstract anger	Prolonged rage
Anger against disease	Anger against helpers
Crying	Collapse
Fear	Anxiety
Fulfilling an ambition	The impossible "quest"
Realistic hope	Unrealistic hope
Sexual drive	Despair
Bargaining	Manipulation

It is important to note that some responses will obtain for the patient an immediate short-term decrease in distress, but will store up trouble in the long term. Denial, once again, is a useful example. If a form of chemotherapy, for example, has a low chance of success (and thus a high chance of failure), a patient might say something such as *Well, we won't even think about the treatment not working*. This may decrease the distress temporarily. However, as will happen in most cases with this therapy, when the treatment does fail, there will come a point at which the patient (and family) have to face that outcome. They may then find it much more difficult to make useful plans in an atmosphere of deep disappointment, disarray, and perhaps despair.

There is a useful analogy here in simple home economics. If an individual has very little money in the bank but decides to use a credit card to finance a big spending spree, there will be a temporary rise in the standard of living as the person lives "off the card." However, this will be followed by a major deficit when the credit card bill comes in, and the lowering of the standard of living at that point is usually much harder to bear and accommodate.

As professionals, therefore, we should try to ask ourselves *What will happen next if the patient (or family) continue on this path*? In other words, we should try to decide not only whether or not a certain response is helping the patient at this moment, but also whether or not it is storing up trouble for the patient later on. To some extent this prediction may be difficult to make, and may depend greatly on the professional's clinical judgment. No matter how difficult it is, this is always an important assessment to attempt, and may make a significant contribution to the future support of the patient.

DISTINGUISHING THE FIXABLE FROM THE UNFIXABLE

Thus, the first criterion in assessing the patient's reactions is social acceptability. The second criterion is adaptation: is this reaction helping the patient to adapt to the circumstances or not? The third criterion is (for maladaptive responses) fixability: if this particular response is not helping the patient, can we intervene to reduce the distress or not? And if we cannot intervene successfully ourselves, are there other professionals who could improve the situation?

Sadly, we have to face the fact that there is some distress that cannot be alleviated, and from which patients cannot (or will not) be rescued.

> **Case History:** The patient was a woman in her mid-seventies who had recurrent breast cancer when she first came to the clinic, dissatisfied with what she was hearing from her previous medical oncologist. She had slowly progressive chest-wall recurrence with no distant metastases. The chest-wall disease covered a wide area and caused sero-sanguineous discharge as well as mild itching and irritation. However, the patient was a fastidious dresser and put great store by her physical appearance. She stated at once that she had accepted

the bad news and was ready to die but could not tolerate loss
of appearance and the inconvenience that the discharge
caused. She had an unmarried daughter who was a devoted
helper, but whom she dismissed as "incompetent." (Curiously,
the daughter half-jokingly agreed: *By my mother's standards I'm
useless.*)

The problem: The patient was exceptionally difficult to please.
The pain was intolerable, but the side effects from even low
doses of analgesics were insufferable. She wanted to remain at
home for as long as possible, but could not tolerate her daughter's low standards of housekeeping. She wanted to maintain
her social life at the local bridge club, but could not stand the
way her friends expressed their sympathy for her plight. Every
agency that became involved in her care (social work, psychology, visiting nurses, homecare, and domiciliary palliative care)
caused deep disappointment and became the focus for more
complaints and frustration.

First reaction: Perhaps the most immediate option would have
been to transfer the patient's care to another medical team. Another option may have been to lay down the law and insist on
very limited communications and not listen to any complaints.

Second thoughts: The patient was actually extremely angry.
She was angry at her complete loss of control and impotence
over her illness, and the inconvenience it was causing. Underneath the anger, contrary to her statement, she seemed to be
very frightened of dying but was unable to admit to that fear.
She expressed her anger in terms of dissatisfaction with the
medical and nursing services, but she was, in essence, "happy
being unhappy." After two or three unsatisfactory interviews,
the care team stopped trying to fix the problems, and set aside
some time (not a lot) to let her air her complaints. All that was
needed was to allow her to list her complaints, and (by not re-
coiling, or rejecting her) to reassure her that the team would
still support her despite her (acknowledged) complaining manner. Although the content of her conversation hardly altered at
all, she began to smile and, in some ways, began to accept
more of her situation, although her list of unfixable problems
remain unaltered.

Practice Point: Do not try to fix the unfixable. Accept it.

In reviewing this history, by what criteria can one decide if a problem is fixable or unfixable? Again, this will depend to some extent on clinical judgment, but the most useful diagnostic signs are the following:

1 Insight: Does the patient have any knowledge of the way in which the behavior is worsening the situation? Does the patient acknowledge the problem if you point it out?
2 Motivation: Does the patient have any desire to alter the behavior?
3 Negotiating abilities: Are there steps that the patient is able to take to modify the behavior pattern?

If the answer to all these questions is "no," then the problem that you are assessing is probably unfixable, and it may not help for you to use your time and energy trying to fix it. If that is the case, as it was with the patient above, then simply supporting the patient by giving a limited quantity of time and attention – despite the unfixable problem – is probably the best option.

If you cannot decide. It often happens that, for various reasons, it is not possible to decide whether a situation is fixable or not. The professional may feel too close to the patient, or too inexperienced, or too upset or angry. Whatever the reason, if there is any doubt about the fixability of a major aspect of the patient's situation, you should get a second opinion. The most valuable source of second opinions varies with local resources. You may have ready access to a psychology department with psychotherapists, psychiatrists, or social workers. If such services are not available, you might be well served with an opinion from another physician, a nurse who knows the patient, or a chaplain or (with caution) a relatively objective family member. A second opinion offers a new perspective on the situation that can often significantly alter your plan of management, particularly if your relationship with the patient has become stuck.

In the practice at the Toronto-Bayview Cancer Centre, approximately two-thirds of the referrals made to the psychologists are for second opinions on this issue. Of those referrals, in two-thirds of the cases some aspect of the patient's situation can be improved to some extent.[54]

Ground Rule: If you think a problem is unfixable but cannot be sure, ask someone else.

CONFLICTS – SOME GENERAL HINTS ON COPING

Conflicts between doctors and patients or families are not rare when the patient is doing badly or the future looks bleak. The emotional temperature is high, the patients are frightened, and the professionals are being challenged. While all parties (including the patient) apparently share the same objective ("doing the very best for the patient") there is occasionally major disagreement about what "the best" actually consists of.

All of us experience conflicts with patients or relatives, and most of us hate confrontations. Any guidelines that are offered here are the counsels of perfection – somewhat like the signs that say *In the event of a fire – Remain calm*, which is good advice and easy to follow at any time other than when there is a fire. However, even though it is difficult to remain calm during a doctor-patient conflict, there are some guidelines that may, at least, stop the conflict from escalating.

Perhaps the most important guideline of all is this: don't forget the basic rules. The greater the conflict, the more important it is to stick to the basic rules of interviewing ("prepare/question/listen/hear/respond") and the six steps of breaking bad news.

Ground Rule: The more difficult the situation is, the more important it is to stick to the basic rules.

In addition, here are some further hints for helping you cope with conflicts.

Try to take one step back
In most such conflicts, the professional finds that he or she is not neutral, but is emotionally involved in the relationship in some way. This emotional involvement is likely to cloud judgment and to influence the professional's ability to make sound clinical decisions. Although these are difficult influences to counteract, it is sometimes possible to try to "take one step back" and define both

the patient's emotional state and the professional's. Here is an example from one of the authors' (R.B.) experience:

> **Case History:** "A young intelligent woman with early breast cancer was already on a low-fat, high-fibre diet, but wanted details of what vitamin supplements she should be taking to decrease her chance of recurrence. Current research provides no evidence that vitamins play a role in recurrence, and I said so several times. She persisted."
>
> **First reaction:** "I actually felt very impatient, and wanted to say *Look, I've already told you four times, there's not a shred of evidence that diet makes any difference – forget it and eat what you like!*"
>
> **Second thoughts:** "I tried to adjust for my feelings of impatience by taking a step back. The patient clearly wanted to hear that dietary change influenced the outcome of breast cancer. Why? On reflection, it was obvious that the patient wanted to exert control over her disease. Accepting chemotherapy (which she did) was a wise decision, but it gave her no personal control over the disease or treatment, whereas altering her diet did. At the same time, I felt that if I were to agree with her statement that dietary changes influenced outcome, I would be endorsing something that I felt was untrue. In the end, I used an empathic response that acknowledged her desire to control the disease (*It must be very hard for you to have this disease and not to be able to control it or the treatment*)."
>
> **Practice Point:** "Taking one step back" during an emotional conflict means trying to assess the patient's emotional stance, and your own.

Describe your own emotions – Don't display them

As part of the same process, you should try to understand what emotion you are feeling, and then try to describe it to the other party instead of displaying it.

In the case of the woman we have just detailed, if the physician found that he was still getting irritated (which is what happened in this case!), instead of saying

> *Look, I've already told you four times, there's not a shred of evidence that diet makes any difference – forget it and eat what you like!*

(which would have been a display of the emotion), the following response decreased the temperature of the conflict instead:

> *I'm really sorry to sound impatient about this, Mrs. Brown, but I've told you the facts as we know them today – vitamins don't affect the outcome of breast cancer. I'm afraid I cannot go on repeating it, but those are the facts.*

Like the *Remain calm* notices, it is easy to observe this rule at any time other than when you are feeling a strong reaction of your own. However, if you can keep a watch on your own emotions, and try to describe them rather than display them, you will certainly improve the chance of resolving a conflict without bad feelings on both side.

Try to achieve a mutual definition of the area of conflict

Sometimes it is impossible to do anything other than to "agree to disagree." In the relationship between a health care professional and patient, this may be a very important element, and is often the only way of resolving a conflict. The objective should be to define as precisely as possible the area of disagreement so that the boundaries of that area, at least, are agreed on by both parties.

Often this approach may help to resolve the emotions that go into the conflict, if not the conflict itself. In the example above, the conflict was clearly definable as a difference in attitude. It was possible for the physician to show sympathy with the patient's viewpoint and to state that he or she would not prevent her from adding vitamins to her diet (advice that would not have been enforceable anyway). At the same time, it was not possible to provide a medical endorsement of any vitamin supplementation. Both parties were satisfied with this definition of the differences and were able to continue without rehashing the argument at each visit. Had this process not been attempted, the argument would have recurred at each visit, or else both parties would have refrained from mentioning the subject for fear of reopening old wounds, in which case the unresolved conflict would have made ordinary clinical communication very difficult.

Try not to be pushed too far from the truth
The problem for professionals with emotional interlocking during a conflict is that we lose the ability to make the best clinical decisions. As we have already seen, patients are dissatisfied with us if we completely ignore their personal traits and personhood. However, we are equally likely to get into difficulties if we respond entirely to the personal characteristics of the patient and get carried too far from the clinical facts of the patient's medical problem. This is a matter of a delicate balance, and it is important. When we have an emotional investment in our relationship with patient (whether it is supportive or antagonistic), we tend to respond to the person (in other words, to the quirks of that particular personality) rather than to the whole situation (which comprises the disease plus the person and the personality). Frequently this involvement results in our being pushed too far from the basic facts or truth of the situation. One example is the way in which we may be tempted to respond to an overanxious patient with over-reassurance and overoptimism. We shall be seeing several other examples in the next part of this chapter.

In general, it is important to try to look at the overall clinical picture. Try to avoid reacting to the conflict itself and instead try to act on your clinical judgment as you would if the conflict did not exist.

> **Ground Rule: In the event of conflict, try to act (on clinical judgment) and not to react (to the conflict).**

SECOND OPINIONS

Whether or not there is a conflict, patients may request (and have the right to) a second opinion. Most of us feel a little defensive when a second opinion is requested and, particularly early on in our careers, feel that our competence is being judged. However, we may have no option, other than recognizing those feelings once they arise. The objective of a second opinion is for the patient to obtain corroboration or refutation of what she or he has heard from you – and you should not stand in the way of that process.

Sometimes, the patient or relative is involved in what is really a form of displacement behavior, and focuses on the activity of "shopping around" as a means of avoiding the facts of the situation. We shall deal with that response in the next section.

In most cases, however, a second opinion is one of the options that are available to all patients in all circumstances except life-threatening emergencies, when there is insufficient time. We have to accept the right to a second opinion as a fact of clinical life.

Specific reactions

The objectives of this section are threefold:

- to assist in *identifying* some of the many types of patients' reactions to bad news;
- to attempt an *understanding* of the root causes of those reactions; and
- to demonstrate some of the *options* that are available as the professional responds to the patient.

There is no chance that this book can achieve either a definitive or a complete description of all possible reactions and the techniques involved in dealing with them. Clinical experience is simply too variegated and slippery to be pinned down in a few pages. There is always something new, and something you have not previously thought of. (As Hippocrates noted, *Life is short, the art long, experience treacherous, judgment difficult.*) After a combined experience of nearly thirty years of breaking bad news, the present authors are still hearing new things, seeing new angles, and meeting new dilemmas (ours and our patients') almost every day.

Second, as already mentioned, human beings can experience several emotions simultaneously. You will commonly see mixtures of different responses in your patient's response to bad news, and the following section can only show some of the ingredients of those mixtures. The more of them that you subsequently recognize in your patients' responses, the more thoroughly you will be able to understand what is going on.

Finally, the following sections deal with patients' reactions. Sometimes those reactions are strong emotions; sometimes they are modes of behavior that can arise from one of several different emotions. Because we intend this book to be a practical guide to what happens most frequently in bad-news interviews, we have not divided this section into "emotions" and "behavior," but will make this distinction clear for each section separately.

DISBELIEF

If it is truly unexpected, bad news is almost always difficult to take in. Hence, disbelief is a very common first reaction to bad news. We all use phrases such as *I don't believe it* in daily life for minor setbacks and surprises, and the phrase shows that disbelief is something we regard as appropriate for major news. You should therefore expect some element of disbelief in most people with whom you share bad news. The essence of disbelief is, basically, *I am having difficulty taking this information in (but I'm trying)*. (This contrasts with denial, which can be summarized as *I will not take this information in*; although, of course, there is a grey area between them and a precise definition of the boundary is not possible.)

Patients express disbelief frequently, and do not intend to provoke an argument with you, but merely to register the fact that they are having difficulty taking the news in. Frequently, there will be evidence of their acceptance of the news through their actions, decisions, or other statements. The combination of stated disbelief with actions and plans that show acceptance is quite common. Your response will be more helpful to the patient if it is based on an understanding of the difficulty of accepting the news (rather than your responding to the overt – spoken – denial). In other words, do not have an argument over the facts with the patient; respond to his or her difficulty in acceptance.

Scenario: A 40-year-old man who is a keep-fit fanatic, except for his smoking, develops lung cancer (picked up on routine CXR). You say *The X-ray shows a tumor in your lung.*

Patient says: *But I run marathons.*

You might respond:

CLOSED QUESTION
Do you think being fit means you can't get cancer? (1)

HOSTILE RESPONSE
Look, you're just going to have to face it – you've got cancer. (2)

OPEN QUESTION
How does that make you feel? (3)

EMPATHIC RESPONSE
It must be very hard to accept a serious illness when you feel so fit. (4)

(1)   Most of us would be tempted – at some stage in our careers, or on certain days at *any* stage in our careers – to respond with something like this, particularly if the patient is aggressive or noisy in protesting how fit he is. This particular closed question is factually correct – you are reminding the patient that being fit does not exclude the presence of lung cancer. However, although you are medically correct, you are omitting recognition of the emotion behind the patient's statement, which is disbelief. This particular closed question is likely to be followed by hostility, and the patient will certainly form the impression that you are ignoring his personal reaction to this devastating piece of news.

(2)   This hostile response is just that. It is certainly true (in some respects and at some levels) that the patient is going to have to face the facts. However, a hostile response will not help him face the facts, but merely remove you as a potential supporter. Open questions and empathic responses, although they do not force confrontation of the facts at the outset, will actually prepare the patient for facing them. Ordering him to do so will not.

(3)   You are on safe ground with this open question. All that the
        open question is really saying is *It is permissible to talk about
        your feelings.* It is quite likely that the first reaction to this
        question will contain some hostility (for instance, *How do you
        think I feel?* or *How would* you *feel if it were you?*), but you
        have established yourself as someone who wants to listen, not
        as someone who wants to tell the patient what to feel. Particu-
        larly if you don't know the patient well, this response is a safe
        option.

(4)   The empathic response here identifies the cause of the diffi-
        culty (that is, how hard it is to take this news on board) as
        disbelief, which is, in itself, attributable to the discordance be-
        tween the way the patient feels (fit) and the nature of the ill-
        ness (serious). This response seems quite simple (which it
        really is), but the central feature of the response is that you are
        not responding to the expression of disbelief. In other words,
        you are responding to what the patient feels, not what the
        patient says.

SHOCK

"Shock" in the common usage of the word (as opposed to the
medical usage, which means hypotensive circulatory failure) is a
form of behavior that is not difficult to recognize. However, it is
extremely difficult to know how to respond to it and how to help
and support a patient going through it.

The central feature of shock is behavior that shows failure of
functioning and, in particular, failure of decision-making caused
by being overwhelmed or overloaded with emotion. People in
shock "don't know what they are doing." They have difficulty in
making decisions, they may act as automatons, or they may have
difficulty in performing simple actions at all. (There was a superb
example in Costa-Gavras's recent film *Missing.* A father, played
by Jack Lemmon, finds out his sone has been killed and as he
leaves the building cannot find his way down a staircase – a near-
perfect representation of shock causing failure of simple decision-

making.) Shock can be caused by many different emotions (such as fear, anger, or sadness) as well as by bad news. It is useful to think of shock not as an emotion in itself, but as behavior indicating a degree or intensity of emotion with which the patient is not able to cope. The load is too much for the patient to bear while still operating normally. Shock is therefore a measure of the severity or depth of the emotion, rather than a separate emotion in itself.

Mental dulling

While the more extreme and rarer manifestations of shock are not difficult to recognize, heavy emotional loads may commonly produce lesser (but still significant) effects on mental processes and thinking. Patients (and family) going through any form of emotional crisis or pressure may suffer from dulling of their ability to think clearly, make decisions quickly, or remember things. These symptoms are so normal that as professionals we may not even remark upon them, but many patients are disturbed by their apparent loss of concentration and may suspect that they have a (new) mental problem as well. Simply pointing out to the patient that this mental dulling is quite normal may provide considerable reassurance.

Manifestations of shock

Some patients may make very dramatic or florid gestures as symptoms of shock in an interview, or at traumatic moments in the course of the disease (recurrence of a cancer is, for example, a particularly traumatic event). One woman walked rapidly back and forth in the room saying loudly *Oh no, oh no, oh no, oh no;* another patient fell to her knees and shouted loudly *Sweet Jesus, don't let this happen.* In both instances it was possible to respond by using an empathic response (as in the next example), after allowing the patients some minutes to express the depth of their feelings (although I had to ask the patient who was walking up and down to sit down after a couple of minutes because it was not possible to talk to her while she was on the move).

Perhaps the commonest symptom of shock is silence. The patient simply is unable to speak or respond to what you are saying. The following illustration offers some options.

Scenario: A young woman with intermittent neurological symptoms has just been told that she has multiple sclerosis.

Patient says nothing, but sits in silence.

You might respond:

CLOSED QUESTION
Would you like me to arrange physiotherapy for you? (1)

HOSTILE RESPONSE
Don't you have anything to say for yourself? (2)

OPEN QUESTION
What are you thinking about right now? (3)

EMPATHIC RESPONSE
This must be overwhelming for you. (4)

OTHER OPTIONS
You might elect to say nothing until the patient speaks again. (5)

(1)   This closed question demonstrates the point I made earlier about closed questions: they can be used by the health care professional in order to avoid painful issues. A patient who says nothing after receiving bad news cannot be thinking of nothing. By filling the silence with a pragmatic question, the doctor is hoping to avoid discussing the emotion which was so painful to the patient that she could not speak. Note that there is nothing intrinsically wrong with this (or any other) closed question: what is wrong here is that the closed question is being used to avoid a painful (and therefore – from the patient's perspective – important) subject.

(2)   Although you might not think so, it is relatively easy to become irritated by patients who say nothing. If you have not been shown how to respond to a silence, the very fact that you don't know what to do next may make you irritated. Once you realize that the best way to end a silence is by concentrating on the emotion that caused it, you will feel less hostile.

(3)   This open question is the "textbook" psychotherapeutic response to a significant silence. By saying this you are indicating that you are prepared to listen to what comes next (which does not, of course, mean that you have to know the answers – merely that you are able to listen to the questions).

(4)   With this empathic response, you are telling the patient that it is permissible to feel overwhelmed by bad news and that the feeling of being overwhelmed is not unexpected (and by extension not "abnormal"). Personally, I find this a very useful response when a patient seems stunned into silence.

(5)   Attentive silence (indicating by body language and nonverbal cues the willingness to listen) may allow the patient to express a deep-seated concern (see chapter 3).

DENIAL

Case History: A cardiologist developed central crushing chest pain that did not resolve with rest. There happened to be an ECG machine at home, and his son who was also a physician did an ECG that showed an infarct. The patient was most upset, and said *It can't be an infarct, I'm chairing a committee meeting this afternoon.*

The essence of denial is the patient's refusal to take on board the bad news, expressing the genuine belief that the news is not real or is a mistake. Another physician colleague reported that he rang the pathologist involved in his case twice – at home – convinced that his slides had been mislabeled and that he did not have prostatic carcinoma. He said that he had a feeling of complete certainty that a mistake had been made, and that the feeling did not fade for several weeks. (This feeling is not unique to one receiving bad news concerning illness, and has been experienced by many of us who have ever in our careers failed an exam!)

In the case of that physician, the denial involved all levels of the patient's perception – at the time of diagnosis there was no part of his mind that entertained the idea that he might have prostatic cancer. The denial "went all the way down." In many cases, denial does not involve all levels, and while the patient is using denial at the overt level of communication, there is already a strong subconscious suspicion, or fear, that the bad news is correct. It is at this point that denial and disbelief shade into each other. This was the case with Mrs. Geraldson (see chapter 4), the woman with ovarian cancer who said *If it's cancer, I don't want you to tell me*. When, later on, she said *Oh well, I knew it was cancer anyway* she was showing that the previous denial did not go all the way down, but that at some level below overt awareness she accepted the diagnosis.

Denial can also be expressed in impassive "irrelevant" behavior, by which a person blocks out the bad news. The following is an example contributed by a colleague:

> A man answers his door on a Saturday morning to a police-man who tells him his wife has just been killed in a motor-vehicle accident. Whereupon the man, without displaying any visible response to the news, proceeds vigorously to paint his house. When his son-in-law arrives several hours later, the man is still hard at it, ignores his visitor, resists interruption from the task, and finally bursts into tears and begins to relate the news of his wife's accidental death.

You may not see irrelevant behavior quite as overt as that, but similar reactions, although less intense, are not rare:

– A husband, sitting with his wife while the physician describes the latest bone scan, suddenly begins to turn the pages of a magazine (without reading them), and will not look up even on direct invitation.
– A patient, at a time of intense emotion, suddenly gets fascinated by her own necklace.

Apart from the overt signs of denial, you may pick up other clues from the patient. A patient may, for instance, start talking about long-term plans (a prolonged university course, or a long-term investment in a business, for example) when there are indications that those plans are not realistic. The approaches set out below may be useful whether the patient's denial is overt (*You're wrong*) or subtle (*I'm enrolling for a PhD course*).

What then is the central element of behavior expressing denial, and how can you best help the patient get beyond such behavior? The central element of denial is a subconscious defense mechanism, functioning to protect the ego, to block out the bad news, and to stop it from penetrating and damaging the patient's view of the future. The way to respond to denial, therefore, is to respect the protective nature of it, and to realize that denial is a normal response to overwhelming threat. Further, you should demonstrate that you are allowing the patient the freedom to deny the bad news until she or he is psychologically ready to deal with it head on.

Here is an illustration of a few of the options available to you in responding to denial at the time of diagnosis.

Scenario: A patient with mild cough and pleuritic pain has just had a bronchoscopy: the biopsy shows small-cell lung cancer. He tells you that he wants to know the diagnosis, and you therefore tell him.

Patient says: *Doctors make mistakes!*   (*)

You might respond:

CLOSED QUESTION
Do you believe we've made a mistake? (1)

HOSTILE RESPONSE
Not this kind of mistake! (2)

OPEN QUESTION
What is it that makes you feel this is a mistake? (3)

EMPATHIC RESPONSE
It must be hard to accept this coming out of the blue. (4)

(*)   Note that the patient's response is not disbelief (as it was with the patient who said *But I run marathons*) but denial, which leaves you no room to maneuver (or so it appears). The patient is not telling you (overtly) that he does not believe he has lung cancer. He is stating that you are wrong and that he does not have the tumor. This response is more likely to spark off a defensive reaction in yourself.

(1)   This closed question is the first step in an escalatory conflict. You are the professional; he is the patient. You can, of course, prove (at a rational level) that he has lung cancer, but the patient's reaction is not simply a rational response; it is a symptom of emotional turmoil. Therefore, to respond to the rational portion of it and to ignore the emotion will separate you from the patient.

(2)   This hostile response is something we are all tempted to use quite often. It is, of course, true – mistakes of this type are extremely rare. However, the patient is clearly having some form of difficulty believing the diagnosis, and you have to cope with his response. Reminding him that you are not making a mistake (which is true) is to ignore his main emotion, and that ignoring causes the damage to the relationship.

(3)   This open question is a better response than the closed question or the hostile response. Depending on the particular patient, it may lead to the patient articulating his denial (something like *I just can't believe it – I feel so well*), which would lead you into adopting a supportive role. However, it might not achieve that end. For instance, the patient might move into a series of rational reasons in an attempt to prove that the diagnosis is wrong. If that happens, you have not made things worse, but you have not moved forward into dealing with the patient's emotion. Therefore, though this open question is unlikely to do harm, it may not do much good.

(4)   The empathic response here achieves three main objectives. It tells the patient that you are aware how difficult it is (*It must be hard ...*); it acknowledges that it is difficult for him to accept the news because he feels well (*... out of the blue ...*); and it also sidesteps the issue of a medical mistake by referring directly to the emotion at the root of the patient's response.

If the patient still insists that you have made a mistake, you have already told him that you know it is difficult to accept the diagnosis. Having said that, you may suggest to him that you can review the histology – as a means of helping him accept the difficult news, not as a defensive (or aggressive) manoeuvre to prove to him that doctors are infallible. You may also want to stress that it takes time to come to terms with this diagnosis, and that further visits will be needed to achieve that.

Often denial occurs at the time of diagnosis, as a part of the patient's initial response to bad news. Sometimes, however, denial can be prolonged, and may be maintained over a period of time despite continuing evidence that the patient's medical condition is deteriorating. This is currently a more common phenomenon because of the widely held belief that a positive attitude influences the course of serious diseases. There is a harmful side effect, which is the consequent belief that "negative thoughts" (for instance, making plans for what to do if the patient gets sicker) will hasten the patient's deterioration. This belief spurs some patients and families into maintaining a continuous shield of denial in the hope that shutting out the negative thoughts will prolong good health. This type of late or prolonged denial can isolate the patient and be difficult to respond to.

Case History: A woman of 35 came to our hospital in Toronto in grave condition. She had been diagnosed a year previously with carcinoma of the cervix, and had received radiotherapy. She then developed recurrence and after only two courses of conventional chemotherapy went elsewhere for alternative-medicine therapies. After persisting with one alternative practitioner for six months she had then flown to Mexico. By this time she was so ill that the Mexican clinic refused to treat her, and she had flown back to Toronto and to our hospital (which happened to be closest to the airport). She was cachectic, had edema to the mid-abdomen, was in early renal failure, and was

three or four weeks away from death. When she was asked
what she made of the illness, she replied *Everyone else has
made a mess of this, and you're going to fix it.* When asked if she
had ever thought of what she would do if this was not possible, she (and her husband) said that they had never for a moment thought of that, at which point she burst into tears.
First reaction: The patient had a perception of the situation
that was very far from reality, and was clearly distressed by
her denial. It would have been tempting to confront this denial
directly and say *Look, you have to be real about this – this disease is going to kill you very soon, and we cannot stop it.*
Second thoughts: It was important to keep in front of her the
possibility that therapy might not work. It was agreed that the
medical team would do what they could for her, if she and her
husband would consider what they would do if therapy was
ineffective. She became more overt about her desire not to talk
about the future, and it was agreed that specific subjects would
not be discussed. Simultaneously, she stopped talking about
"cure" or "fixing the disease." As long as the prognosis was
not discussed overtly, she remained content (far more so than
when she first arrived) and continued talking easily on all
other subjects with ward staff and family until her death.

Denial in this case was really manifested as excessive hope. While
some element of hope allows all of us to get through the day
whatever our circumstances, there can be side effects of denial
that is manifested as excessive hope. Cassell expressed this most
clearly in his analysis of the different types of hope,[55] and perhaps
what he called "hangman's hope" is best considered as a subcategory of denial. In his analysis of the patient's motivations, he
used the following analogy:

This morning I found myself running to catch an airplane. I
was running along the concourse towards the gate at the exact
time that the aircraft was meant to take off. But I continued
running, hoping that I would catch the plane. Was that hope
justified? Sometimes aircraft are delayed in take-off (this one
was, and I caught it). But would I have been justified if I was

running towards the gate four hours after take-off time? Or twenty-four hours?

Furthermore my ticket was the kind I could change. I also had a timetable of other flights in my pocket. But what if I had had a non-changeable ticket and if I had never even thought of or contemplated alternative flights?

Surely, some hopes are realistic and some are not. If you have alternative plans and timetables and if running does not cost you too dearly, then nothing is lost by trying. If however, all your plans are based on catching that plane and you're already too late, then your hope is of a different sort. I call that hangman's hope: it is the hope that a prisoner has that when he is hanged the rope will break. It may not be a helpful way for a person to face a threat.

As we have already discussed, denial at the early stages of hearing bad news can be a normal and useful method of taking the news on board in small chunks – when it appears to the patient that otherwise it would be overwhelming. Prolonged or late denial (as in the last case) increases distress (one of the causes of that patient's tear) and needs detailed negotiation and cautious handling.

DISPLACEMENT

There is a reaction to bad news that is relatively common, but for which there is no totally satisfactory descriptive word in current use. Quite often patients *divert* the emotions and the emotional energy that have been precipitated by the illness into an action or activity. This activity may help them cope (that is, it may be adaptive), or it may not, but the key feature is that the activity releases the emotions or energies that originated with the bad news. The word "displacement" has many meanings (in Freudian psychology the phrase "displacement behavior" is used to describe a person refocusing his or her emotions onto a person or object distant or distinct from the true source of the emotions). In its common usage, however, it usefully describes the way in which patients divert their emotions after hearing bad news.

Case History: Shortly after hearing the diagnosis of recurrent carcinoma of the ovary Mrs. Miller, a 40-year-old woman, and her husband undertook considerable research into the illness, reading many recent articles and telephoning several major experts all over the continent. Undertaking this activity made them both feel better and more equipped to cope with the bad news. They felt that their questions were more focused, and their strategies and their participation in decision-making more informed.

Assessing the value of displacement activity: We must make it clear that identifying something that the patient is doing as displacement activity does not imply criticism or denigration. Displacement activity can often be a major part of the patient's coping mechanisms. The activity that the patient undertakes may be very valuable in assisting the patient to cope with the illness. It may become a symbol or a metaphor for the illness and allow the patient to resolve several emotions or conflicts. The activity may even help not only the patient but also friends or family or society at large, and may offer something of lasting worth.

The criteria by which you should assess the value of any displacement behavior are those you use in any reaction to bad news: is this response adaptive or maladaptive, and (if it is maladaptive) will intervention improve things? Thus, a displacement task that reduces the patient's distress (whatever the nature of the task) should be reinforced, and one that increases a patient's distress should become the subject of a dialogue between you and the patient.

The emotional content of displacement activity: Note also that we are describing activity that has an emotional content. The patient undertakes the activity while expressing one or more emotions, which may include enthusiasm, anger, frustration, sadness, or denial among others. This is quite different from the scenario (described in the section on denial) in which a man painted his house energetically after hearing that his wife had been killed. In that situation, the man used the activity (house-painting) to block out the bad news and to prevent himself from expressing any of the emotions precipitated by it. In displacement activities, the person performs the activity (whether it is reading medical journals, keeping a diary of events, or something quite separate such as housework or a hobby) while expressing the emotions released by the bad news. Displacement behavior comes in all forms and sizes, and may be related to the medical bad news or unrelated to it.

Displacement behavior *related to the bad news* is very common. Frequently, the activity is related to gathering information about the disease, or recording daily medical events (often in the form of a diary or proposed book), or making sweeping changes in diet or life-style. All of these may serve an adaptive function or a maladaptive one, depending on whether they aid the patient in adjusting to the new medical circumstances.

Displacement behavior that is *unrelated to the precipitating cause* is also common. In daily life we have all done things like this (haven't we?), doing the dishes angrily in the middle of an argument, or getting out and mowing the lawn with more energy than usual after having a piece of bad news or disappointment. The activity can be usual for the patient or unusual: such as developing a new interest in a sport or hobby, or reviving an old and neglected interest or project. Whatever the activity, if it is undertaken as a result of the bad news and if the patient uses the activity to release the emotions that have been triggered by the bad news, then the activity is serving a replacement function for that patient. Depending on the circumstances it may play a useful role in resolving some of the pent-up emotion.

Sometimes the displacement activity becomes a major goal or obsession for the patient, and may come to be a quest in the patient's life. There are other ways in which a goal or objective may become a quest for the patient; we should therefore look at these next.

THE QUEST

Some projects expand to occupy a major and central position in a patient's life after she or he hears bad news – the activity takes on the proportions of a quest. For these purposes we shall define a quest as a project that is more unusual in size, scope, or nature than any undertaken by the patient before the illness. A quest may originate in one of three main settings:

- as a form of *displacement* behavior (when it may be either adaptive or maladaptive)
- as the fulfillment of a previously held *ambition*
- as the expression of *denial*

1. *Displacement behavior*

Adaptive disreplacement behavior – The "really useful project": A patient may react to medical bad news by creating something of lasting value to herself or himself and the community at large. The project may be a work of research, artistic creation, or education. The cardinal signs of a really useful project are the signs of an adaptive response: the patient is better able to face of the situation and expresses less duress and distress. The patient does not deny or avoid the medical situation, but is assisting in her or his own support. Often this will be accompanied by an increase in participation in the decision-making about their care. When these signs are present, you should reinforce the value of the project for the patient and you should emphasize the adaptive role of the activity. To adapt the old adage:

> **Ground Rule: Some patients, when life hands them a lemon, learn to make lemonade.**

Maladaptive replacement behavior: On the other hand, a project can occupy a patient's attention and then preoccupy it, replacing all other activities and increasing distress. A well-known example is the often-quoted one of Dr. Franz J. Ingelfinger, late editor of the *New England Journal of Medicine*. When he developed carcinoma of the esophagus, he searched through hundred of articles and sought (or was offered) dozens of expert opinions on the best treatment. It seems that his distress became more and more marked until a friend of his said *What you need is a doctor.*[56]

The central point of that example is that the patient can help himself or herself by participating, but not by taking on the role of the doctor as well. Dr. Ingelfinger's distress was the sign of the maladaptive response: he needed someone to give him overt permission to delegate some of the responsibility for his treatment to another person, the doctor. Participating in the decision-making should – and must – be encouraged: but taking it over entirely is likely to produce the distress mentioned above. Here is an example of some of the options available in that situation, some of which will allow you to respond without diminishing or demeaning the patient's involvement.

Scenario: Patient has newly diagnosed ulcerative colitis.

Patient says: *I've done all my reading and here's what I want you to do.*

You might respond:

CLOSED QUESTION
Do you think I don't know enough about the subject? (1)

HOSTILE RESPONSE
*Do **you** think that I don't know enough about the subject?* (2)

OPEN QUESTION
Tell me what you're most concerned about? (3)

EMPATHIC RESPONSE
This must be very worrying for you – there seems to be so much to know and so many options. (4)

---

(1)   This closed question (which may be asked quite calmly) takes the dialogue straight into the area of the physician's competence. This response – phrased as a question – is a response to the perceived challenge by the patient: *Who knows more, me or you?* In responding like this, you take the focus away from the patient and his or her motives, into issues of medical facts. This may make it more difficult to come back to the patient's feelings later.

(2)   The same words can carry different emotional force – and this
        is an example. Here the same sentence conveys considerable
        aggression, motivated by a defensive reaction to a challenge in
        a very sensitive area (professional competence). The same com-
        ments apply to this response as to the closed question above.
        This is a response to the overt content of the patient's reaction
        and ignores the motives for that reaction.

(3)   As is usual with an open question, you are on reasonably safe
        ground. Most patients who are deeply involved in a quest will
        not necessarily be aware of what is driving them and will reply
        to this open question with something like *Well, I'm really con-
        cerned about the response rate in the Wisconsin study*, in which
        case you are no further ahead, although no damage has been
        done. Occasionally, a patient will "let you in" and reveal the
        motive behind the activity.

(4)   With this empathic response you are giving the patient permis-
        sion to feel confused – and also encouraging him or her to be
        the patient, not the expert.

---

2. Fulfillment of an ambition

Sometimes a quest is an ambition (unrelated to the illness) that
the patient has nursed for many years before the disease occurred.
If you find that the ambition is long-standing then you can certainly encourage the patient to see whether there are feasible steps
by which it can be fulfilled. The key here is that the ambition
should predate the disease. If that is the case, then the quest is
consistent with the patient's premorbid state and is part of the
person not part of the reaction to the disease.

3. Denial

The quest motivated by denial can be recognized because in order
for the project to be completed, the prognosis would have to be
wrong. In other words, the project is a way of the patient saying
*The doctors must have got it wrong – and I shall prove that by com-
pleting this project.*

Case History: A man of 35 telephoned a physician whom he had never met to say that he had just been diagnosed as having motor-neurone disease (Lou Gehrig's disease) and had three years to live. He wanted to enroll many physicians and other patients in a large fund-raising project with the stated objective of finding the cure for motor-neurone disease before he died of it.   *(Continued below)*

The quest motivated by denial may be massive and ambitious (as was this man's) or more personal (such as undertaking a three-year PhD course or making long-term business investments). Often the patient presents the project to the family and health professionals almost as a challenge: *You say I won't live long – I say I will. Now you would have to be very cruel if you want me to drop this idea, so perhaps you'll back down.*

Like all denial, a quest driven by denial can serve a useful function if it later allows the patient to accept the situation. Many patients change the nature of their quests or what they gain from them as the disease progresses, as happened with the patient with motor-neurone disease.

Case History continued: As the patient's disease progressed, he at first became bitter and angry and then withdrawn. However, by this time his fund-raising efforts had brought him into contact with a very wide range of people who supported him in every imaginable way. As he realized that he would not be able to finance the cure for motor-neurone disease, his role in the group changed and he allowed himself to receive support instead of being the exclusive dynamo of the group. His fundraisers took on the additional function of a support group, which made all the participants feel more worthwhile.

Perhaps the most important feature of responding to any quest is to take a step back.

Ground Rule: With a quest, don't look at what the patient is doing for the quest, look at what the quest is doing for the patient.

FEAR AND ANXIETY

Fear of ill health is normal. In fact, if one of your patients shows
no fear when hearing some serious news, your first reaction should
be *Has this patient understood what I have been saying?* Of course,
there are the rare patients who can face any medical reverses with
perfect equanimity, but by and large some degree of fear is so
common that we should be on the alert if we see no evidence of
it at all.

Fear vs Anxiety

While we can all agree that fear of ill health is normal, there is a
great deal of confusion about the words we use to describe that
feeling. The biggest confusion surrounds the words "fear" and
"anxiety." Are there any differences between those two emotions?
If there are, what are they and do they matter? Before we discuss
an approach to helping patients through their fears and/or anxieties it is important to try to reduce the linguistic confusion as far
as is possible. As we shall demonstrate, there are differences between fears and anxieties, and they have some implications for
the way we approach these emotions.

Linguistic confusion: The first problem is that in daily life we
use "fear" and "anxiety" almost interchangeably. Both words describe an emotional state of dread or apprehension (which may
be accompanied by a variety of physical signs of sympathetic-
nervous-system overactivity, including tachypnea, tachycardia,
hypertension, dry mouth, "butterflies in the stomach," and so on).
However, we quite often use "anxiety" as a euphemism (a socially
acceptable circumlocution) when we really mean "fear" but do
not want to say so. For instance, a politician might express publicly
some "anxiety" about the outcome of a debate, but would never
confess to feeling fear. Anxiety is acceptable for public consump-
tion, but fear is not, because the word anxiety has a far more
clinical and accurate sound to it. When we don't mind saying that
we are afraid (among friends at a horror movie, for example), we
would not use "anxiety." If we heard someone say *I saw the film*

Nightmare on Elm Street *last night and found it highly anxiety-provoking*, we might suspect that the person was a psychologist or was perhaps trying to sound like one.

Differences between fear and anxiety: Despite our common use of the words interchangeably, there do seem to be two main differences between fear and anxiety. First, fears tend to be specific and are usually triggered by a specific object or event, or by the thought of that object or event. Anxieties, by contrast, tend to be more diffuse and usually extend beyond the objects or thoughts that trigger them, sometimes having no triggers at all.

In addition to the difference in specific triggers, it also seems (from our general use of the words) that fears are usually more acute, coming on rapidly with the trigger and usually fading rapidly when the trigger is removed. Anxieties tend to be more chronic states and, even though their onset may be acute, usually take longer to resolve, even after any triggering event has passed. This may be a useful way of thinking about these two states, even though there are clearly gray areas between the two, and the placing of any border is, to some extent, subjective.[57] For the sake of completeness, we should add the definition of *phobia* as a fear that is disproportionate to the situation, inexplicable, beyond voluntary control, and leading to avoidance of the feared situation. *Panic* describes an acute state, a sudden surge of acute terror, accompanied by somatic symptoms, during which the patient has great difficulty with coherent thought and decision-making. The key feature of a panic state is, therefore, the patient's inability to make reasoned decisions – the emotional state has overloaded the patient's rational capabilities.

Apprehensive states – A practical approach
However, the definition and labeling of a psychological state of apprehension is of less importance than a practical approach to alleviating it. Perhaps the most important aspect of dealing with a patient's fear or anxiety is finding out what specifically the feeling is caused by. Then one can attempt to provide the relevant aid, whether it is information, psychological support, or medica-

tion, or a combination of all three. The following are the four most useful steps in dealing with such states:

1 Identify the *causes* or roots of the fear, anxiety, phobia, or panic.
2 *Acknowledge* the existence of the patient's feelings (at the initial stage, without expressing your own judgment on whether the extent of feeling is appropriate to the emotion or not).
3 Offer the most relevant *information.*
4 *See what happens:* if the information reduces the intensity of the emotion, continue to provide it; if it does not, then offer empathic support for the patient; and if the problem is severe and continued, obtain a second opinion from a psychologist or psychiatrist.

Let us examine those steps in greater detail, one at a time.

Step 1. Identify the cause: You can do nothing for your apprehensive patient until you have shown that you are ready and able to listen to his or her feelings sufficiently to identify the source. Any form of premature reassurance before that is done will be ineffective, and will not reduce the intensity of the emotions.

Step 2. Acknowledge the existence of the patient's feelings: This, as we have mentioned, is the second ingredient of the empathic response. The process of identifying and acknowledging may, itself, reduce the problem somewhat in some cases. Here is an example in which the patient has a very specifically triggered fear.

Scenario: You have a patient with unstable angina, and have just suggested that he have a coronary angiogram to determine the extent of his atherosclerosis.

Patient says: *No. I can't go through with an angiogram: my tennis partner died during one of those two years ago.*

Note: Death during an angiogram occurs in less than 0.5 percent of cases on average.

You might respond:

CLOSED QUESTION
Do you think that's going to hap-
pen to you? (1)

HOSTILE RESPONSE
Oh for goodness' sake – the mor-
tality of the procedure is less than
half a percent! (2)

OPEN QUESTION
What worries you most about all
this? (3)

EMPATHIC RESPONSE
That must have been very dis-
tressing for you – have you been
thinking it might happen to you?
(4)

_____

(1)   Note that this closed question is not "wrong," but is a legiti-
       mate tool to help unravel the patient's state. This is not a ques-
       tion aimed.at proving the superiority of the doctor's knowledge
       (such as *Do you know the mortality of the coronary angiogram?*
       might have been), but is a way of eliciting the relevance of the
       past experience to the patient's current perception of his state.
       (See also chapter 3.)

(2)   This hostile response is not a rare one in clinical practice. After
       all, you know (as a professional) that the morality rate of 0.5
       percent is very low – 199 out of 200 patients survive the pro-
       cedure. It is factually correct, but it ignores the emotional state
       of the patient (which contains the fear that he is the one out of
       two hundred who will die – a fear based on his past experi-
       ence of the unexpected death of his partner). Even if this re-
       sponse is used in an attempt to be "heavily reassuring" it will
       not achieve this. Giving reassurance requires acknowledgment
       of the patient's reaction first. This response ignores the pa-
       tient's reaction altogether.

(3)   The open question gives the patient permission to talk about
       his reaction (as does the closed question in this instance).

(4)   The empathic response in this example goes further than does
       the open question. It recognizes the fear of the patient and tells
       him that the doctor expects the patient to be frightened by the
       previous death – and, therefore, that this fear is not abnormal.

Note that you are not simply reassuring the patient – in fact there is no such thing as simply reassuring the patient. Nor are you allaying his fears (the mortality rate of angiography is still 0.5 percent, and neither you nor the patient knows whether he will or will not be that one in two hundred). Once you realize that you are listening to the patient and giving him permission to feel what he is feeling (whether or not you would feel the same emotions yourself in his position) you are halfway to understanding this part of the approach to fear and anxiety.

As you try to identify the patient's fears and anxieties about illness, it is quite useful to have some framework or classification in mind. Although the commonest source of fear is probably the basic fear of the unknown, the major sources of fear vary considerably from individual to individual and with the consequences (real or perceived) of the illness. We have already seen in chapter 2 how the various fears of dying are also individual; the more the professional is able to identify the fears expressed by the patient, the more easy it becomes to acknowledge the patient's feelings.

Step 3. Provide information: Having acknowledged the existence of the patient's feelings and having gone some of the way towards diagnosing the main objects of those feelings, you can go on to provide whatever specific information seems relevant to the situation. Obviously this depends on the extent of your own knowledge and on your role in the team.

Step 4. See what happens: If the information provides some relief, and the intensity of the emotion is diminished, then you have achieved something. You should continue to provide further information as the patient asks for it and needs it. If the patient is receptive to what you have to say, but the information does not seem to help (that is, if the emotion is information-resistant), do not keep repeating the same information, hoping that one day the patient will feel less apprehensive. You can continue to empathize with the patient's feelings, but if the patient's symptoms are severe or prolonged, then you should get some help (from a psycho-therapist, psychiatrist, or other specialist). Here is an example in which a patient's anxiety was totally information-resistant.

Scenario: The patient is a young woman with carcinoma of the ovary. Her disease is in complete remission, but there is an 85 percent chance that it will recur within the next five years.

Patient says: *I can't do a thing — all I think about all the time is the cancer coming back.*

You might respond:

CLOSED QUESTION
Do you have any trouble sleeping?
(1)

HOSTILE RESPONSE
Oh for goodness' sake — you're absolutely fine. Stop complaining and get on with your life. (2)

OPEN QUESTION
What are your main worries?
(3)

EMPATHIC RESPONSE
It must be awful for you being constantly worried about recurr-ence. (4)

FALSE REASSURANCE
Please listen to me — it's not going to come back, and that's that. There is no need to worry. (5)

---

(1)   With a medical-history style of question (even though it is aimed at a symptom associated with anxiety or depression) the doctor is attempting to change the subject. He or she may also be trying to get the patient to see that "things aren't that bad really" (that is, if sleep is not disturbed, perhaps the anxiety can be classified as trivial). This approach is unlikely to suc-ceed. The patient needs to have the anxiety noted; if it is imply ignored the patient will fell unsupported. Once the anxiety is

noted, the patient will feel differently about the physician –
even though she may admit to the physician (as this patient
constantly did) that the anxiety was unfixable.

(2)   This hostile response is a direct expression of the physician's
        irritation. It can only lead to the patient feeling rejected and to
        a worsening of the problem.

(3)   The open question is a prelude to the physician noting and ac-
        knowledging the existence of the patient's anxiety.

(4)   The empathic response takes the interview straight into the
        area of the patient's feelings. It does not (and perhaps cannot)
        offer an instant remedy for the anxiety state, but id does estab-
        lish between the two of you that the anxiety is a legitimate
        subject for discussion. You may want to stress the fact that
        uncertainty is always painful but is a fact of this particular
        medical situation (*so let's see if we can find ways of dealing
        with it ...*).

(5)   This response – although proffered with the good intention of
        reducing the patient's anxiety – is dangerous. False reassurance
        will lead to considerable panic and loss of trust if the disease
        recurs (as, in this scenario, will happen 85 times out of 100),
        and you will then be unable to help because you were clearly
        wrong in your prediction. In fact, the patient may subcon-
        sciously push you into over-reassurance, and it is important to
        resist it as firmly as you can, staying as close to the truth as
        possible. Nothing else will sustain your relationship in the
        longer run.

The dangers of over-reassurance

Perhaps the most important precaution here is taken from response
option (5). Over-reassurance is the most dangerous option because
it pushes you further away from the true situation as time goes
on. The trouble is that the more anxious the patient, the stronger
will be your own desire to alleviate the distress and the greater

your temptation to over-reassure. Here is another example taken from a past (disastrous) experience that happened to one of the authors (R.B.):

> **Case History:** "The patient was a man in his fifties with chronic Guillain-Barré syndrome who had been bedridden for several months. His neurological improvement was negligible and we had agreed not to offer any prognostic prophesies (or guesses). On a ward-round (which, as the resident, I was conducting while my senior staff physician was away) I found a very slight improvement in his leg power, and he asked me (as he often had before) whether he would be out of hospital before Christmas. Rashly, I answered *Yes, I don't see why not.* I thought I might buy some peace and encouragement for him, but in fact I had really given in to the patient's desire to hear good news, even if it was false. The effect was disastrous. The patient clung to my reply, and reminded everybody of it on every subsequent ward-round (*But Dr. Buckman said I'd be out by Christmas* ...). It needed weeks of support to undo the damage and the disappointment that I had caused."

It may be worth emphasizing as a

> **Ground Rule: When the patient is extremely anxious, do not overcompensate by being over-reassuring. (Another example of the rule: "act, do not react.")**

But perhaps the final word on fears and anxieties should be to stress the importance of referral for the patient who is not making progress. Whatever your own seniority and experience, if the patient's condition is not improving, think seriously of obtaining some outside assessment.

> **Ground Rule: If things do not improve, get some help.**

ANGER AND BLAME

Anger (hostility or rage) is another emotion that is common is breaking-bad-news interviews. It may be subtle or overt, and it may be directed against one or more of many targets – quite often the health care professional is the primary target. For the reason it is helpful to have some understanding of the anger that patients may feel. It is also useful to have thought out a few techniques of responding to it without being overwhelmed or provoked into an angry response yourself.

It is worth trying to classify the targets of anger (see the following table): in facing an emotion – and particularly anger – familiarity and recognition make it easier to maintain your own equanimity, and therefore respond supportively. It is less difficult to respond to, say, a patient's rage against a particularly heathy young cousin (or even yourself) if you know that this kind of resentment is common. Recognizing it early on makes it easier to phrase an empathic response, for example, and thus to maintain a supportive role in the face of potential conflict.

Furthermore, the realization that there are a large number of different targets of anger (as listed in the following table) reduces your own desire to regard someone else's anger as "aberrant" or "pathological" – thus decreasing the temptation to make a judgmental (and thus unhelpful) response.

Blame is really a subcategory of focused anger: it implies anger directed against some specific person or agency, and (depending on the medical facts of the situation) may be either appropriate or inappropriate.

A "ROUGH AND READY" CLASSIFICATION OF PATIENTS' ANGER

ABSTRACT ANGER
(unfocused)

Against the disease
against symptoms; against "death sentence"; against disability, loss of freedom

Against loss of control and powerlessness
against inability to determine life-style/movements; against dependency on relatives, medical team

Against loss of potential
against loss of chance of fulfillment; against loss of future hopes and aspirations in career, relationships, family

Against laws of nature/randomness
(depending on patient's belief system) against random biological events; against unfairness (one of the causes of "Why me?")

ANGER AGAINST SPECIFIC ENTITIES
(focused)

Against self
causal anger (if patient feels he/she has caused own disease – either appropriately or inappropriately); against body or biology (resents specific failure of body); against opportunities missed (regrets concerning specific events or relationship); against own attitude (the downside of believing that a positive attitude improves the outcome)

Against friends and family
against their health (resentment of the fact that they are healthy); residual anger from old rifts or family feuds; against having to be the recipient of advice, charity and sympathy; causal anger (belief that friends or family contributed to causing disease – appropriate (e.g., AIDS, other sexually transmitted diseases, lung cancer in passive smoker, etc.) or inappropriate; against abandonment or distancing (relatives or friends withdrawing from patient)

Against medical and other health professional teams
blaming messenger for the news; against loss of control, which now resides with doctors/nurses; resentment that medical team members are healthy; against communication gaps (not listening/cold/insensitive/uncaring); against management decisions (should have found it sooner/treated it differently)

Against "outside forces"
directed at workplace/occupation (appropriate or inappropriate); directed at environment/home (appropriate or inappropriate); directed at socio-economic/political forces

Against God
against abandonment (*He has forsaken me*); against perceived vindictiveness (*Divine Retribution*); against apparent poor return on faith and religious observances over many years

Here is an example in which the anger is ostensibly directed against a previous physician:

Scenario: Patient has had epigastric pain for two months, diagnosed after a perforation as a gastric ulcer.

Patient says: *That other doctor said my pain was nothing serious – now I've got an ulcer. I'm going to sue that idiot!*

You might respond:

CLOSED QUESTION
Didn't he even order a barium meal? (1)

HOSTILE RESPONSE
Listen, if you're planning to sue that doctor, you're certainly not going to get any help from me. (2)

OPEN QUESTION
What are you feeling now? (3)

EMPATHIC RESPONSE
You sound angry that this wasn't picked up earlier. (4)

---

(1)   At this point you have no idea whether the previous physician did anything inappropriate or even whether any action would have made a difference. There is a great temptation to use a closed question to ascertain the facts of the case; however, that is unlikely to achieve anything. Asking the patient for details of previous management will only give you the patient's perception of what happened. This is extremely important in understanding the patient's emotions, but it is not a valid way of deciding whether or not the previous doctor's management was at fault. The patient is demanding a response, but you cannot offer a judgment on the previous doctor's management based only on the patient's perception of it. Also, by saying "didn't *even* do a barium meal" you are already taking sides and joining the patient in blaming the previous doctor. Without any factual information, this is a dangerous step to take. First, the patient will use your authority in amplifying the resentment towards the previous physician, and may be even more tempted to go to court with your apparent backing. Sec-

ond, a patient who feels this way towards previous doctors will shortly feel that way about you. You therefore have to find a way to acknowledge the emotion that the patient is feeling without commenting one way or the other on the merit of the medical case. This can be achieved by either the open question or the empathic response cited here.

(2)   We all hate being challenged professionally. Very often, a patient's criticism of our profession hurts us personally. This kind of response shows what many of us feel deep down inside – it is an aggressive-defensive response. However deeply it is felt, it will cause deterioration of your relationship with the patient, because it is a personal and to some extent unprofessional response from you, inviting further criticism of the profession. It can only cause the patient's anger to escalate.

(3)   The open question is deceptively simply here. It completely sidesteps the issue of whether or not the previous doctor was a fault and switches the entire focus onto the patient's feelings. The response therefore sends this message to this patient: *I don't know anything about your previous doctor's management, but I'm here to care for you. Your feelings are important – let's talk about them.* This is an example of how an open question directed at the patient's emotions can rarely lead you astray. The patient's response is likely to be explosive – much of the anger, resentment, and blame may come out. However, you have asked to hear about it and you are, to some extent, in control of the situation instead of being caught up as an ill-informed witness in a lawsuit.

(4)   It seems almost too simple to acknowledge the emotion that the patient is expressing and no more. However, when the emotional temperature is high, you should stick to what you know. Your response may well trigger further anger (*Well, of course I feel angry ... wouldn't you*), but as with the open question you will not be the target of it, and you will not be inflating the patient's anger. You can then move on from the "shoulds and oughts" of the past to the things that must be done about the current situation.

Anger can also disguise fear. Patients may feel that it is not socially permissible to express fear, but that it is permissible to express anger. This is another reason why you should always try and find out the root cause of the anger – if it is fear, then it will not be assuaged by counteragression, but only by giving permission for the fear to be expressed.

Another type of anger is theological – anger directed against God. If that is where the patient's anger originates, you will almost certainly require a chaplain's (or other religious equivalent's) help to deal with it.

> **Practice Point:** One further note about responding to anger. Human beings seem to be programmed to decrease their anger when it meets a submissive response. Body language that moves away from counteraggression helps to diffuse a patient's anger. When a patient is angry, it is always worth trying to keep your head lower than the patient's. A useful technique is to have the patient seated upright on the examination couch, while you sit on a chair or stool. It is interesting to note how difficult it is to maintain anger when the target of it is sitting below you.

GUILT

Guilt is not an easy reaction to define. In clinical terms it seems to have three essential components:
 – It is an emotion that is self-focused or *self-directed*.
 – There is *self-blame*.
 – There is an element of sorrow or *regret*.
(In this context, we are considering only the guilt experienced in reaction to illness – a sense of guilt about a crime, say by a burglar or embezzler, is a mark of potential future improvement, and absence of guilt or remorse is the hallmark of the sociopath or psychopath.)

Although this may be a somewhat contentious view, in clinical practice it seems clear that, with rare exceptions, guilt about an illness is almost always maladaptive and hardly ever useful to the patient. It is true that, sometimes, the struggle to overcome a sense of guilt may call upon hidden resources within the patient and may later reveal unsuspected strengths or values, but the guilt itself is, with few exceptions, another problem and never part of the solution.

The exceptions are those situations in which a sense of guilt gives the patient the necessary incentive to modify his or her behavior in a way that improves the outcome. This is almost entirely limited to secondary prevention; if a patient has a heart attack or an episode of chronic bronchitis, giving up cigarette-smoking will decrease the chance of recurrence. If a sense of guilt tips the balance between ceasing smoking and continuing, then it might be argued that the guilt has some secondary value to the patient in increasing the incentive to modify future behavior, though it could still be said that the emotion itself is not of primary value.

Guilt (like blame) may be based on appropriate or inappropriate data, depending on the medical circumstances. A surprising number of patients with multiple sclerosis, for example, feel that they have brought the disease on themselves (a conclusion for which there is no evidence whatever), whereas with a self-inflicted disease such as small-cell lung cancer (97 percent of the cases involve smokers) many patients do not perceive or cannot acknowledge their own role in causation. From the physician's point of view, the "appropriateness" is not the central issue – the guilt itself is part of the patient's problem, whether or not it is based on medically valid data.

> **Case History:** The patient was an unmarried physician in her early forties when she presented with an early-stage breast cancer. She worked excessively hard as a family practitioner. Unexpectedly, she spent most of the first three or four interviews crying. For much of the time she castigated herself with guilt at having ignored the breast lump (for perhaps a month or two). At first, we tried to point out that her tumor was a small one, the lymph nodes were negative, and her prognosis was relatively good. However, she continued to cry and call herself "stupid, stupid, stupid."

First reaction: It was tempting to appeal to her physician's understanding of the situation, and to remonstrate with her about the prognosis. However, she was extremely angry with herself and also felt very guilty.

Options: We decided that the guilt itself was unlikely to be a fixable problem. We simply responded to her crying by staying with her and acknowledging that she felt guilty even though (as a physician) she knew that she had not jeopardized her medical condition. Although she never allowed discussion of the guilt as such, over several months it became less extreme in its expression.

To stress it once more:

> **Ground Rule: Guilt about the illness is almost always useless to the patient (though it may occasionally have a secondary value in affecting future behavior).**

Here are some of the options for dealing with a patient expressing guilt feelings, set out in our usual format.

Scenario: A smoker is diagnosed with lung cancer.

Patient says: *I wish I had never smoked. Now, I'm going to die and I deserve it.*

You might respond:

CLOSED QUESTION
How many years have you smoked? (1)

HOSTILE RESPONSE
You should have thought of that years ago, and done something about it. (2)

OPEN QUESTION
Tell me what you are feeling. (3)

EMPATHIC RESPONSE
It must be very painful thinking it's your fault that you got lung cancer. (4)

(1)   The closed "medical history" type of question is a way of
        avoiding the central issue here (that is, that the patient feels
        that he has caused his own disease) and sends a message to
        the patient that the issue of his guilt feelings is not to be dis-
        cussed.

(2)   The hostile response is never helpful to the patient. Any re-
        sponse on the lines of *I told you so* – however much we may
        feel we want to say it – puts us on the side of the patient's
        problems (in this case, adding to the feeling of guilt) instead of
        on the side of the problem-solver.

(3)   The open question here says a very important thing; that is, *I
        think your feelings are a legitimate topic for our discussion – tell
        me more.*

(4)   In this empathic response, you identify the emotion that the
        patient is feeling ("painful") and you identify the source of the
        pain as guilt ("your fault"). At the same time, you give the pa-
        tient permission to discuss the feelings, and you have not
        made any comment about whether or not the disease is the pa-
        tient's fault. You can then move on to the current clinical situa-
        tion and discuss the things that the patient and clinician can
        undertake and plan in these new circumstances.

HOPE, DESPAIR, AND DEPRESSION

Hope and Despair

The word "despair" comes from the Latin, meaning loss of hope,
although we use it commonly to imply a major and acute loss of
hope. (Curiously, the more chronic state of hopelessness is surprisingly rare in chronic illness – hardly more frequent than in the
general population.[58])

   We tend to use the word "despair" to describe an acute lowering
of mood, and in many respects, hope and despair are opposite

sides of a seesaw. They are two emotional reactions to the same facts, and it should not come as a surprise to see patients seesawing back and forth between moods of hope and odds of despair. If a patient has, for instance, a disease with, perhaps, a chance of recovery of 30 percent, that person might feel one day that she or he will be among the fortunate 30 percent and that recovery will occur. The next day she or he might feel that she or he is among the unlucky 70 percent and will not recover. The facts have not changed, but the emotional coloring of the patient's perception of those facts has flipped from one state to another. The two states are mutually exclusive.

Despair is a heavy burden for patient and professional, and there is often great pressure to lighten the load (for both parties) and to reduce the distress of despair by promises or contracts that later cannot be fulfilled (as discussed in the section on anxiety above). In responding to despair you should try to adhere to three principles:

1. Do not promise anything you cannot deliver
If the despair seems to be unwarranted by the medical facts, then you may reinforce the facts. If, however, the possibilities are serious, then do not backtrack and change the medical facts when confronted by despair (see "Fear and Anxiety," above – this is similar to the to the guideline on anxiety "do not respond with over-reassurance," and is another example of "act, don't react"). You should, even under pressure, stay as close to the reality (even if it includes uncertainty) as is possible, stressing that you will do whatever you can do and will not abandon the patient.

2. Always allow the patient to express his or her despair
Do not panic during this ventilation, but try to allow the patient to express the deepest feelings (within reason).

3. Reinforce the fact that the patient will not be abandoned
Your relationship will continue.

Depression
The word "depression" is used to describe a more chronic state of lowering of mood. It is known that some people have a pre-

dilection for affective disorders (disorders of mood) that may be bipolar (the old-fashioned "manic-depressive disorder") or uni-polar (intermittent "endogenous" depression). In patients with these disorders, episodes of depression may be triggered for no apparent reason. However, even in patients with no preceding history of depressive disorders, depression may be provoked by the threat of serious illness, and probably occurs in up to 20 percent or more of all patients with major illness,[59] particularly cancer.[60] Most of us would regard a serious threat to health or life as a legitimate trigger for depression of mood in any individual, but it does not matter whether we think the threat is appropriate or not. What matters is the diagnosis of the depressive state and its treatment.

As regards modern nomenclature, the most recent classifications of mental disorders separate depression from a group of conditions termed "adjustment disorders." To put it as a simple paraphrase, an adjustment disorder is "what you'd expect, given the circum-stances," and it may be accompanied by a variety of moods, such as "adjustment disorder with depressed mood," "adjustment dis-order, with anxious mood," or "adjustment disorder with dis-turbance of conduct," and so on. Depression, by contrast, is (approximately) "more than you'd expect given the circumstances" and is accompanied by the symptoms listed below. To a large extent, this whole book is about people going through adjustments, and for our purposes it may be less useful to attempt to delineate the borders between adjustment disorder with depressed mood and depression than to recognize the symptoms of depression (as listed), because those symptoms indicate an illness[61] that responds to therapy.

Whatever the premorbid state of the individual (whether or not he or she has been prone to depressive periods before), the most important elements of your approach to depression should be the following:

1. Make the diagnosis: Depression is a disorder with well-rec-ognized physical symptoms (see following table). With any patient facing bad news, be aware of the physical symptoms of depression and look out for them. They may be common – symptoms of true depression may occur in up to 30 percent of patients with breast cancer, for instance, whatever form of surgery they have had, and whether or not there is any recurrence of the disease.

SYMPTOMS OF DEPRESSION[62]

---

1 Depressed mood, or irritability
2 Markedly diminished interest or pleasure in almost all activities
3 Significant weight loss or gain, or decrease or increase in appetite
4 Insomnia or pypersomnia
5 Psychomotor agitation or retardation
6 Fatigue or loss of energy
7 Feelings of worthlessness or excessive or inappropriate guilt
8 Diminished ability to think or concentrate, or indecisiveness
9 Recurrent thoughts of death or recurrent suicidal ideation

For a diagnosis of "major depressive episode" at least five of the above symptoms must have been present during a two-week period, and at least one of the symptoms must be either (1) depressed mood or (2) loss of interest or pleasure.

---

2. Identify the depression for the patient: This is a remarkably useful manoeuvre. It is easy and helpful to list the symptoms to the patient and formalize the diagnosis (*You're getting loss of sleep with early-morning wakening, and loss of appetite and libido. Those are all symptoms of depression, which means that there are two problems going on – the illness that we are dealing with and this second problem, which is depression and which is quite common in these circumstances.*) Very often the patient is relieved to know that the symptoms make sense and that the condition is common (and therefore legitimate).

3. Be prepared to treat it: Having made the diagnosis, try and assess the severity of the depression. It may (rarely) be life-threatening and the patient may be seriously contemplating suicide. If the patient expresses suicidal ideation, and you are not in a position to assess the likelihood of suicide (although it is not a common event,[63] even in cancer patients[64]), obtain a psychiatric referral.

> **Ground Rule: Don't ignore any talk of suicide. Obtain the assessment of someone experienced in the field.**

If the symptoms of depression are not severe at that moment, it is often useful to tell the patient that the condition can be treated if it does not resolve in a short time (perhaps two or three weeks). Antidepressants (for a period of a few months) are probably underused in these circumstances because so many professionals think that depression is "expected and normal" after hearing bad news, but in fact treatment for depression usually produces a major improvement.[65] Depression may indeed be expected – as may pain after a broken leg – but that does not mean it should not be treated.

> Ground Rule: Severe depression related to physical illness is usually treatable.

OVERDEPENDENCY

It is both flattering and frustrating for a health care professional when a patient becomes heavily dependent on her or him. In some respects, this is a side effect of supportive care: the patient is stating (or, more usually, demonstrating) that the professional is perceived as a supportive individual and can be relied on. This response is flattering to one's sense of professionalism, but overdependency is also dangerous to the patient, to the patient's coping strategies, and to your relationship.

The diagnosis of overdependency is not clear-cut, and there will always be a strong subjective element to it. All relationships between patients and professionals contain some element of dependence, and what is overdependent behavior to one physician may be seen as appropriate or compliant behavior to another, or even manipulative or seductive behavior to a third. Perhaps the best criterion by which to distinguish overdependency from the mainstream of doctor-patient relationships is that overdependency decreases the patient's abilities of self-determination – in other words, the patient tends to delegate decisions about his or her condition that would previously have been his or her own to make. In itself, this is not deleterious to the patient (as long as you, as the professional, are willing and able to assist with the decision-making), but it usually leads to disruption later. There is commonly an initial period of mutual respect and admiration during which you are perceived as more and more helpful; but this is often followed by the patient's disenchantment as your limits of toler-

ance are exceeded and you can no longer give unlimited time and
energy to the patient's demands.

The key to handling overdependence is first to try and separate
the patient's needs from her or his demands, and second to try to
agree on a contract that involves bilateral responsibilities. The first
step is not always easy. The patient is likely to be highly motivated
in presenting all demands as essential needs. Some of these will
indeed be needs and, of these, it will be in your power to meet
some but not others. It is important for you to state this fact as
clearly (but gently) as possible, and as early as possible. You can
state overtly what you will try to do, but there is an enormous,
almost palpable difference between *I will try to ...* or *I will do my
best to ...* and the promissory *I will ...* When the patient is overdependent, resist the temptation to buy temporary peace from
importuning by overstanding your capabilities or powers (yet another example of "act, don't react"). As in responding to anxiety,
when the patient is heavily dependent:

**Ground Rule: Don't be pressured into promising the moon
(unless you happen to be able to deliver it).**

By attempting to define the patient's needs and stating as clearly
as possible how you will attempt to meet them, you are then,
implicitly, defining the remainder of the patient's requests as demands. Your turning down any demand will cause the patient
some pain; nevertheless, it is the only way to avoid an increase
in overdependency. The situation can be clarified, with minimum
distress to the patient, by establishing a contract between the two
of you. You need to stress what you will do (and can do) and, at
the same time, stress to the patient the activities that you cannot
and will not do, but which remain the province of the patient.
This obviously requires some delicacy and gets easier with experience, but there are structures of speech that may help, such as:

> *I can monitor the effect on the tumor and I'll tell you
> whether it's getting bigger or smaller, but only you can say
> how bad the treatment is – so I'll rely on you to tell me how
> you feel.*

or

> *That decision about buying the new house isn't one that I*

can make for you. I will tell you at each visit how things are going, but I can't make the decision about the house for you. That's your decision – though I can give you all the information you want as we go along.

Ground Rule: In responding to overdependency, try to reinforce a contractual relationship that increases the patient's sense of self-reliance.

CRYING AND TEARS

Crying is not an emotion, it is a symptom. It can be a symptom of several different emotions – fright, relief, pain, anger, rage, frustration, sadness, despair, depression, love, humor, and many others. Some people are moved to tears easily and will cry when almost any emotion reaches what some would call moderate intensity, while others do not cry even when passionately moved.

Curiously, most people are not very good at coping with the tears of strangers. We know that tears signal distress, but unless the person crying is a friend we usually seem a bit stuck when it comes to giving comfort. The following are the practical steps that I find most useful when a patient cries:

1. Move closer to the patient
Most people feel very vulnerable when crying (as well as feeling ugly and unattractive), and feel even worse if they are rejected or shunned. Depending on what you guess to be the patient's comfort level, move a little closer, or at the very least do not move away.

2. Offer a tissue or handkerchief
This is essential. Make sure you always have tissues available in the office or consulting room. If it happens that there are none, ask the patient if he or she has a handkerchief available – and if not, go and get one! *Nothing else will do.* A tissue or handkerchief achieves four things: (1) it gives the patient overt permission to cry; (2) it gives the patient a means to restore his or her face somewhat (it is impossible to talk normally if your nose is running uncontrollably) and perhaps partially hide it; (3) offering it gives you something to do if you are feeling embarrassed; and (4) it simultaneously brings you into closer proximity to the patient.

3. Touch the patient
If you are both comfortable with contact: the contact can be light and slight (resting your hand briefly on the patient's elbow or shoulder) or more overtly supportive (putting your arm around the patient's should if you are certain this will not be misinterpreted).

4. Try to identify the emotion that is causing the tears
This may be obvious, in which case you can use an empathic response. If the cause is not obvious, you can use an open question (such as *Are you able to tell me what is making you cry at the moment?*).

5. Stay with the patient until things are a little calmer
If you have to leave the room or bedside, ask the patient if he or she wants to be alone – if not, try to find someone (a relative or a member of the team) to stay with the patient for a while. If that cannot be achieved, apologize (which at least tells the patient what you would have liked to do if you had been able).

> **Ground Rule: If the patient cries, offer tissues or a handkerchief.**

Crying as an acute reaction is normal and common. Prolonged, uncontrollable, and unstoppable crying is rarer and more serious. If a patient (or a relative) cries continuously at several visits over a period of time with undiminished pain, then you should seek some help in supporting him or her. The patient may well benefit from counseling and from having "a professional shoulder to unload some of this pain onto" (a phrase that is useful on many such occasions). Even a small number of weekly sessions can help greatly, depending on the circumstances.

> **Practice Point:** If the crying doesn't decrease, get some help.

WHY ME?

Why me? is a response to bad news that seems to be a question but usually is not. *Why me?*, like tears and crying, is a symptom (in this case a form of behavior) that may originate from any of several different emotions.

It is much more useful and practical for you to think of *Why me?* as a cry, and not as a true question. As a cry, it may be an expression of despair, anger, frustration, or guilt. You may not be able to define instantly the major emotion behind the cry or (if there seem to be several) which are the most important ones. If you attempt to answer this response as a direction question, you may lose the chance of ever finding out.

Why me? can be precipitated by specific aspects of the disease or treatment, by general aspects of the illness, or by pre-existing dilemmas in the patient's life or in the family or social relationships. Unless you ask what the specific precipitating factor is, you may respond with an answer that is not relevant, perhaps even unhelpful. To express it as a

> **Ground Rule: When responding to *Why me?* you do not need to answer straightaway – ask first.**

Here are some options:

Scenario: You have just told a young man that he has motor-neurone (Lou Gehrig's) disease.

Patient says: *Why me?*

You might respond:

FACTUAL RESPONSE
We don't know the answer to that – the cause of motor-neurone disease is completely unknown. (1)

HOSTILE RESPONSE
It's always someone – this time it's you. (2)

OPEN QUESTION
Can you try to tell me what you are feeling at this moment? (3)

EMPATHIC RESPONSE
You must be feeling awful hearing this. (4)

---

(1)   I have selected a direct answer instead of a closed question, because it is highly unlikely that you would be tempted to answer an open question with a closed one. You are far more

likely to be pushed into answering with a factual response. If it happens that this is what is bothering the patient (*Did I do anything to cause my motor-neurone disease?*), then your answer will be exactly what the patient wants to hear. The point is that you don't know. If you ask first (see the open question below), then you can follow up with a factual response if that is what is wanted. Again, there is nothing intrinsically wrong with this response; it just may lead you away from an important emotion that the patient is trying to express.

(2)   This response is not intended to be hostile, but is used (and I have seen it used in practice) to stop a philosophical argument with a philosophical coup de grace. *Why not me?* is a state of acceptance that many patients may reach on their own after much thought, and it may have philosophical or theological meaning for that person. However, if you (as a healthy professional) present it to the patient, you not only are ignoring the emotion behind the cry, but also are taking the discussion on to an abstracted level, which will make you appear cold and indifferent.

(3)   Without wishing to appear dogmatic, I must say that this is by far the best response to the cry *Why me?* What you will hear in response to your question will surprise you – the range of emotions that may prompt a *Why me?* is wide. If you find the way I have phrased your question too bald, you may be more comfortable with a preface such as *People may mean several different things when they say "why me?" May I ask you ...,* which may make you feel less embarrassed.

(4)   If it is clear to you what emotion is being expressed by the patient, then an empathic response that identifies that emotion may be perfectly satisfactory here.

RELIEF

Although it may seem paradoxical, or even crazy, some patients greet medical bad news with relief. This happens most commonly when the patient has had a prodromal illness that has been difficult to diagnose or has caused symptoms that have not been believed. A typical example is multiple sclerosis, in which the initial symptoms may be sensory only, with minimal physical signs. The patient is aware that something serious is wrong, but nobody believes the symptoms and the anxiety increases. In this circumstance, despite the bad news of the diagnosis, the patient is relieved that she or he is not going crazy after all. Such a reaction can occur even when the diagnosis is very serious if the patient has had a major pre-existing worry about it.

> **Case History:** Mary R. was a woman of 45 who had had breast cancer diagnosed three years earlier. She received adjuvant chemotherapy, but was extremely worried about the possibility of recurrence, even though she was symptom-free, and was quite demanding in her continuing need for reassurance. She developed back pain in her third postoperative year and a bone scan showed multiple metastases. When she was told of this, she cried (as did her 15-year-old daughter, who was with her). Then she quite suddenly stopped crying and said to her daughter *Well, now we know what we're up against.* Curiously, from that moment on she was far calmer and braver than she had been before the metastases appeared.

THREATS

Patients can rarely control serious medical conditions, and may often search for areas that they can control. Making a threat is often a mechanism by which a patient can demonstrate some level of control over what is happening. The threat may be directed against the doctor (for instance, the threat of legal action or of transferring care), but is quite often directed at the patient himself or herself in the form of a threat of suicide or damage. Of course, all threats are likely to contain some measure of aggression or hostility, but quite often that emotion itself is triggered by the insecurity that comes from loss of control, and the apparent aggression is actually a defensive response. Threats may be expressed with a degree of calm and courage, which makes conversation and discussion very difficult.

The most important things to remember in responding to a threat of any kind are the following:

1. Stay calm

Threats of any kind are very upsetting, and it is easy to become agitated and defensive yourself. If you can, stay calm and try not to enhance the primary gain of the threat by showing that it works. As the phrase goes, *Let them push your buzzer, but don't let them hear the bell ring.*

2. Identify the objective of the threat and acknowledge it

If you do not identify the threat in your conversation, then you cannot compensate for it. It is very important that you let the patient know that you understand the objective of the threat (*I do realize that you might want to find another doctor for yourself ...*) and that you respect the right to hold that feeling (*... and of course you are quite entitled to do that).*

3. Ask the patient to suspend the threat

Threats make two-way conversation difficult. The most effective technique that I have seen for responding to a threat involves simply asking the patient to suspend the threat. (*I find that it's very difficult to talk about the situation while you are threatening to stop treatment. Perhaps we can discuss how you feel first and then, after we've talked about it, if you really want to stop treatment, then of course that is your right.*)

In some ways, a patient may display apparent calm and bravery, and that itself may contain an implied threat (*I'm not afraid of death, so either you do what I say or I'll let myself die*). The patient mentioned in the first part of this chapter (who had a chest-wall recurrence of breast cancer and whose daughter was, in her eyes, inadequate) used the fact that she was apparently ready to face death as a stick to beat both her daughter and her physician. By acknowledging the possibility of death (instead of making promises that death was not at all likely) the physician reduced the power of the threat, while still allowing the patient to talk about her major fears.

Here is an example in the usual format:

Scenario: The patient is a socially isolated 75-year-old lady with glaucoma. She has no past psychiatric history.

Note: Antidepressants are contraindicated for patients with glaucoma.

Patient says: *If you really cared for me you'd give me some pills so I could kill myself.*

You might respond:

DIRECT RESPONSE
I'm afraid I can't do that.   (1)

HOSTILE RESPONSE
Oh for goodness' sake, stop that and pull yourself together!   (2)

OPEN QUESTION
Tell me what you've been feeling.
(3)

EMPATHIC RESPONSE
You sound very depressed about your situation.   (4)

REMOVAL OF THREAT
Can we start by talking about why you feel so desperate?   (5)

(1)   This direct response is factually correct: you cannot give a patient medication for the express intention of assisting suicide. However, it closes the door on any possible dialogue about why the patient feels this way. It's correct, but limiting.

(2)   You may want the patient to pull herself together (whatever that means), but even if that is your objective, telling her to do so will not achieve it.

(3)   A direct invitation to talk about the feelings will not stop any threats of suicide, but will definitely establish you as a listener.

(4)   The empathic response here identifies (and thus validates) the depression.

(5)   This response goes a little further than the empathic response. You are saying *I know you are depressed, but I want to sidestep the threat of suicide for the moment.* Using the word "first" implies you will return to the other content of her statement later.

However, this patient definitely needs help. If you cannot offer her sufficient time and support, then she will benefit from a referral to a psychiatrist or therapist.

To put it all into one

Ground Rule: Threats of any kind make it difficult to behave normally and easily. If at all possible try to appear calm even if you do not feel it, and try to respond to the emotion underneath the threat, not to the threat itself. If you are stuck, get help.

HUMOR

Appropriate humor

Humor is an aspect of human behaviour that, in contemporary society, is either taken too seriously or not seriously enough. At one end of the scale are those who believe that laughter can influence the outcome of serious diseases; by contrast, in conventional medical schools it is not mentioned in the curriculum at all. It seems likely that, among other things, humor is an important behavioral mechanism by which some people cope with the world and put into perspective certain threatening events that might otherwise seem overwhelming. It is possible that humor evolved (probably at the same time as symbolic language) as a means of putting a frame around something that appears to threaten the individual or community. Even today, the commonest subjects for jokes are things that are threatening or frightening and that, in themselves and in reality, are not funny at all. (Why else do we have all those jokes about sexual problems, diseases, death, flying, marital disputes, and in-laws – none of which are intrinsically funny in real life?)

However, humor is not part of every individual's armamentarium, although it is central for some:

Case History: Mrs. Rolls was one of the most genuinely witty and charming women anyone could wish to meet. She had had a mastectomy several years before she first attended the clinic (when she was 63), and she continued to have difficulties with her ill-fitting external breast prosthesis. She once said that she had been swimming the previous day, when her prosthesis fell out of her swimming costume and floated towards the shallow end while she was swimming towards the deep end. Sensing that something was wrong, she had turned and spotted the floating prosthesis and had said to her swimming companion *Ah well, there it goes, doing the breast-stroke on its own.* She was immensely proud of her joke (and rightly so) but, more important, it typified her own coping strategies. When things got bad for her later on, she carried on until the end of her life putting misfortune in perspective with her own humor and inventions, which made her a favorite and memorable patient.

There is no right or wrong about the importance of humor to a patient; it is simply a matter of individual personality – like the importance of food or sex. However, it is very important for us to recognize that humor can be a useful coping strategy for some people and that you may respond to it and reinforce its use.

The word "respond" is used here advisedly – you *cannot* use humor with a patient who does not use it himself or herself. If you decide to "cheer someone up" and start an interview with a joke or a frivolous remark, it is likely that the patient will perceive you as someone who does not take her or his predicament seriously. You will appear to be distancing yourself from the patient's suffering. If, however, the patient makes a joke first, then she or he is showing a desire to be distanced from her or his suffering, and is rising above it. Your response to that humor encourages the process and reinforces the patient's coping.

Ground Rule: When it comes to humor, respond to the patient's humor, don't inflict your own – a pre-emptive strike can go badly wrong.

Inappropriate laughter and humor
However, a word of caution – not all laughter involves humor, nor are all jokes humorous. Some patients laugh when they are tense, and their laughter is misread as an indication of ease.

Case History: Mrs. Stevens, a university professor in her early forties, sought several different medical opinions on the surgical management of her primary breast cancer. She consulted a colleague of mine who recommended Treatment X, with which – he thought – she seemed very pleased. She later complained bitterly that she had wanted Treatment Y and was very upset that this was not recommended to her. In discussing the interview with a psychologist who had also met the patient, it occurred to all of us that this patient smiled more and more intensely when she was angry – a signal that was interpreted by my colleague as approval.

Practice Point: In responding to a patient's laughter (or smiles), be on the alert for discordance – and disparity between the content of the speech and the facial expressions.

Jokes can also give a false signal. Some patients use jokes to present a false impression of their state of bravery or preparedness. You have to try and decide whether, underneath the humor, the patient has actually come to grips with the situation or not. In the case of Mrs. Rolls above, it seemed clear to me that she understood the situation at each stage of her illness, and her behavior did not change. Other patients use jokes as a substitute for coming to grips with the situation, and want you to accept the humor in place of their acceptance of their circumstances. This kind of behavior requires very careful responses from you, and you might well need some advice or help in dealing with a patient who uses humor as an escape instead of a coping mechanism.

SEDUCTION

The "difficult" patient is not always the one who is peculiarly nasty to us; difficult patients are quite often ones who are peculiarly nice to us. In both cases, the motivation is usually fright (fear of the disease) and a desire to be special to the doctor or nurse, and therefore to receive special care. There are two basic methods of obtaining special attention – the carrot and the stick. Seduction (by any method) is the carrot method.

Seduction can take many forms (of which sexual seduction is not the commonest). Perhaps the two commonest forms are gifts and excessive praise. Either of these should alert you to the possibility of future problems. Gifts from patients, particularly around Christmas and if modest, may be regarded as tokens within the normal boundaries of social interaction. Extravagant or lavish gifts pose a real problem for the health care professional. If there is no such thing as a free lunch, there is certainly no such thing as a free gift from a patient. Whether the intention is stated or implied, a lavish gift is a psychological (or actual) bribe and means that the patient expects lavish or special treatment. Those expectations may consist of extra attention (the patient may wish to phone you at your home, see you personally at every visit, or have you do house calls) or guarantees of cure.

> **Case History:** "Mrs. Jackson was a woman in her early seventies who presented with a pleural effusion as the first symptom of her ovarian carcinoma. Her disease responded to therapy and she (and her husband) were very pleased with me but excessively demanding. At one point she thrust several hundred dollars at me and would not take it back when I said it wasn't right for me to accept the gift. I gave the money to the research fund at the clinic and had the receipt made out to her (which removed my overt obligation to her without having to have a fight). However, I suspected that her attitude to me would change dramatically when her disease became chemo-resistant. I was right – a few months after the donation, her disease recurred. She and her family did not accept that I had done my best (and did not recall that I had told them the disease would probably recur). They implied that, having made this donation, she had a right to remain in remission."

Excessive praise has the same effect. If you find yourself being praised in a way that you suspect is out of proportion to your achievement or effort (*You are the best ...*), and particularly if you are compared to the patient's previous doctor, who is now held in disfavor – beware. The same cycle is likely to be repeated. In proportion to the high praise, you can expect expressions of major disappointment and criticism if things go badly for the patient.

How to handle lavish praise or gifts: However rude or churlish it may appear, you should try and remind the patient of the true situation at the time (*Thank you for the compliment – but it's the drug that did the work, and we don't know what the future will bring* or *You really are doing well now, but I honestly don't know how long that will last*). The more overt you are about the transaction that is being carried out (maintaining kindness and politeness) the better. This is another example of the rule "acknowledgment of any embarrassing factor of which you and the patient are aware reduces the embarrassment." You do not have to refuse all expressions of gratitude, but you do have to make it clear that the other end of the bargain (as the patient perceives it) is not in your power to give (*Thank you for the praise/present – I wish I could guarantee your future in return*).

The same technique can be used in any form of seduction or pressure: if you overtly acknowledge the excessive attention (*This is very flattering of you, but ...*), you partly reduce the leverage.

> **Ground Rule: Beware of excessive praise – disaster is usually around the corner. As with responding to a threat, you may neutralize subtle pressures by acknowledging them overtly.**

BARGAINING

A lot has been written about the process of bargaining, particularly since Kubler-Ross identified it as a stage of the process of dying. In the view of the present authors, bargaining is not a stage, but is part of the process of rationalizing the threat of illness and reestablishing some control over the future. One can think of bargaining in this way: the patient fears that the disease may have a grave outcome (for instance, it may prove fatal), but hopes that it will not (that there will be a remission or a cure). Both of these are emotional reactions that are, to some extent, outside the sphere of rationality and beyond the patient's control, either physically or intellectually. By bargaining, the patient may build a rational or intellectual bridge leading away from what he or she fears and towards what he or she hopes for (*If I promise to do X, then the disease will go into remission and not kill me*).

Bargaining can be a useful part of a person's coping strategies and can act as an adaptive response. Sometimes prolonged and unrealistic bargaining (bargaining that increasingly draws the patient further from the true situation) can increase the distress of the situation and become maladaptive. In any event, some people use bargaining and some do not. When you recogniz the process of bargaining, try to assess it in terms of whether or not it is assisting the patient's adjustment, and if it is helping, treat it as you would any other part of the patient's coping strategies.

AWKWARD QUESTIONS

We have selected three questions that most doctors seem to dislike answering. Obviously they are more likely to arise when the disease is life-threatening, but the techniques employed in responding to these questions may be useful in other situations.

How long have I got?

Not all bad news carries an implicit threat of death, but when it does the question *How long have I got?* is probably the single most common question asked by patients or families. Most doctors hate this question for many reasons, including the following:

- Physicians are not good at guessing about the survival of patients and dislike being proved wrong (one study showed that relatives and nurses were better at these predictions – and that the performance status of the patient was as good an index as anything or anybody).[65a]
- Giving an indication of expected survival is an explicit admission of the failure of curative therapy.
- A gloomy prognosis (even if accurate) may lead the patient to seek other opinions in the hope of hearing something more favorable (even if inaccurate).
- The patient and relatives will take particular note of how the physician replies and may well select parts of the answer out of context (*He gave me three months at most*).
- The question may precipitate a difficult conversation about the process of dying with which the physician may feel uncomfortable (see chapter 2).

For all these reasons, the pressure rises when this question is asked – and, for all these reasons, it is even more valuable to stick to the guidelines I have suggested. You should think of the answer to the question an another item of bad news. The objective of your answering this question is a process of aligning, followed by a process of educating. In doing this bear in mind the following principles.

1. Aligning: Ask the patient what he or she thinks the situation is. Try to get a rough picture of what the patient makes of the clinical situation and the risk as explained so far (*What have you been thinking yourself?*). This will give you your baseline upon which you can build.

You should also make sure that the patient is truly asking about survival (it is quite useful to reiterate the question *Do you mean how long do I think you will live?*). In another case, a patient asked her doctor *How long will it be?*, a question that the doctor thought concerned her imminent death. For some reason he asked her what she meant, and it transpired that she meant *How long will it be before I am back at work?* From that starting point much more discussion was required before he could bring her closer to the true situation.

2. Educating: In steering the patient towards the clinical facts, bear in mind the following

> **Two Ground Rules: (1) You have to give the patient the right sort of idea – "the ballpark figure." (2) You have to be aware that your answer will be remembered (possibly inaccurately) for a long time.**

It is most important not to be too far away from the truth when answering the *how long have I got?* question. As we have said, doctors are notoriously inaccurate in their predictions, but nonetheless you do have to give some honest indication of the situation. I almost always use language that gives the patient a reasonably accurate understanding, although it is usually a ballpark estimate or range (*I think it will be several or many months* or *It may be a small number of years, but it is not likely to be many* or *I think the situation is quite serious – we may be looking at several weeks or a small number of months*). Very often a patient will ask *Could it be three months?* or something similar. I always try to avoid hard figures, not because I am cowardly, but because I am likely to be wrong. I usually try to stress the range rather than the single figure (*It's likely to be several months – anything from two or three months to five or six*). The patient may still tell the family *The doctor gave me three months*, but at least you know you have tried.

3. Uncertainty: Uncertainty is one of the most painful aspects of serious illness. Shuttling back and forth between hope and despair has been described by one patient as a "grueling roller coaster" – of which the descent from hope is often the worst part (*It's not the despair – I can cope with the despair – it's the hope that kills me*[66]). It is not possible for the professional to banish the pain of uncertainty, but she or he can reduce its impact by acknowledging it. (*It must be very hard for you not knowing what's going to happen next or when*). It is a good idea to resist the patient's pressure to make more accurate guesses than you are able to make: instead express an empathic response that legitimizes the unpleasantness of uncertainty.

> **Ground Rule: Uncertainty is highly unpleasant. It will help your patient if you acknowledge this fact.**

Am I terminal?
The question *Am I terminal?* is also quite common. One physician (on a witnessed ward-round) once answered that question with a sympathetic shrug and *Well, we're all terminal*. The patient was not pleased, and felt (correctly) she had been dismissed.

One caution in answering this question: ask the patient to state what he or she means by the word "terminal." Some patients mean *I am dying now*, while others mean *I am eventually going to die of this disease*. Without your aligning your answer on the patient's perception and meaning of the word terminal, you may get stuck quite quickly. Aligning can be achieved quite simply (for example, *That's a very important question and I'll try and answer it for you. But first, can you tell me what you're thinking about when you say "terminal"?*).

What will it be like?

When responding to the question *What will it be like?* the process of aligning is as important as it is in the preceding examples. *What will it be like?* almost always contains a desire to discuss (and, if possible, to have answered) the deepest concerns and fears that the patient has about death and dying. You cannot even begin to answer the question usefully unless you find out what the patient is most worried about.

The fears about dying set out in chapter 2 show some of the range of possible concerns; any individual patient may have any (or many) of them. Hence you should regard this question as an opening for a discussion, not a request for a single factual response. Here are some of the possible approaches.

Scenario: You have just told a patient that curative therapy is not working and your objectives now are palliative.

Patient says: *What will it be like?*

You might respond:

FACTUAL RESPONSE
It will probably be fairly slow and you won't suffer too much. (1)

DIRECT RESPONSE
Let's face all that as we come to it. (2)

OPEN QUESTION
Can you try to tell me what you are most worried about? (3)

EMPATHIC RESPONSE
You must be very worried about the future. (4)

---

(1)   For the reasons that we have already mentioned, a factual response might suffice, but you will not have any idea what the patient wants to ask about unless you ask first. You might get stuck quite quickly with this response.

(2)   This direct response is really an evasion. Again, some patients might be ambivalent about wanting this question answered and might welcome the chance to postpone a discussion they think they ought to have but do not really want to. You will detect that if you use the open question.

(3)   As with answering the two previous questions, the open question is of enormous value here. As we saw in chapter 2, the range of worries that a patient might have is wide, and you can perform a great therapeutic benefit by acknowledging the main fears and anxieties at this moment.

(4)   The empathic response is perfectly acceptable here. It is probably a little less useful than the open question, but it will certainly allow and encourage the patient to list his or her main worries.

Sometimes, a discussion of the process of dying can get into too much detail for the patient's comfort, and may increase the patient's distress instead of reducing it. It is always worth remembering that you do not *have* to cover every aspect of the end of life in a single conversation. There will often be a point in these conversations at which is is useful to pause (as in the response *Let's face that when we come to it*) and resume the conversation later. The patient will have received the message that you are available to discuss the issues and you recognize the value and legitimacy of discussing them. Further references on communicating with the dying patient can be found in textbooks and reviews on palliative care.[67]

BREAKING BAD NEWS TO CHILDREN

Children are special in almost every meaning of that word. When it comes to breaking bad news to children – whether it is about themselves or others – you may require special expertise or special qualities of your own. Considerable expertise has evolved in the techniques of counseling children about serious disease; there are entire books written on the subject.[68] In general, as with adults, good psychosocial adjustment for children is associated with early knowledge of the diagnosis and not with concealment or evasion.[69] Although this task usually falls within the province of those professionals with specialist training and skills, there may be unusual occasions in which you are called upon to talk to children without the assistance of an expert counselor. There are several important principles to bear in mind:

1. Have the closest adult relative present if at all possible
Only in the direst emergency should you try to talk to a child (of any age) without the nearest adult next-of-kin present. If at all possible, talk to the adult first and agree on the manner in which the information will be shared with the child. The adult may want to participate (which you should welcome), and may have valuable insights into what will be the most difficult areas for the child. If the adult has no particular warnings, then you can briefly describe how you are going to conduct the interview so that there will be no major surprises.

2. Check your communication level frequently
Children's understanding of the world advances with age and maturity, but there are no guaranteed milestones. You cannot be certain that a child of five will not understand the threat of serious illness or death, or that a child of nine will. More than in any other setting, you must check your communication level frequently and make sure that you are providing information that aligns with the understanding of the child. Pick your language to match the child's questions, and check frequently to make sure your messages are being received.

3. Be ready to repeat things
Children often require repetition of information, not because they are unintelligent but because they need to be reassured that they have understood it correctly. Be prepared to answer the same question frequently; this is often the only way that the child has of assuring himself or herself that you really mean what you say.

4. Understand "magical thinking"
There are several differences between the ways children and adults view the world. One of the most important (certainly as regards breaking bad news) has been called *magical thinking*. This phrase is used to describe the way children tend to believe that their thoughts or actions can magically cause events to happen in the

outside world. One form of this is seen when a child temporarily wishes bad luck on someone (a common example is putting a spell or a curse on someone): if something bad later happens to that person, the child may feel responsible and guilty. Children are thus quite likely to feel personally responsible if someone they know receives medical bad news, and may in some way feel that any anger or resentment they felt about that person has now brought about illness. The same is true of actions that have no relevance to the medical situation. A parent may repeatedly tell a child, for example, to keep his or her bedroom tidy (which most normal children do not). If the parent later falls ill, the child may be plagued with the guilty thought *If only I had kept my bedroom tidy, mum wouldn't be ill now.*

Children rarely express these ideas directly (and very rarely to doctors at the first meeting). It is therefore very important when talking to children to make it clear that the illness is nobody's fault (even if they have not expressed the idea that they have caused it). It is often worth specifying this in detail (*This illness is not your mum's fault, it's not our fault, and it's definitely not your fault. This is just a piece of bad luck, one of the bad things that happen sometimes*).

5. Get professional help as soon as you can
Talking about bad news to children is not an area for the inexperienced or uncertain health care worker. Depending on your position in the team, you may want to find someone who does this often (or ask someone else to do that). If you know the family well, you may be a reassuring additional presence at the subsequent interviews with the ore experienced professional, and you may learn a great deal yourself.

THE SEARCH FOR MEANING

The meaning of suffering is really a philosophical matter for the individual concerned. However, you may become involved in a person's search for the meaning of an illness, and it is all too easy to dismiss that search as fruitless, and to attribute no meaning to the illness other than that of biological accident. This is not an issue that a book like this can answer definitively. However, there are two ways in which the word "meaning" can be used, and they each have different implications for any conversations on the subject.

Some people use the word meaning in the sense of "intrinsic meaning of the illness" – a meaning that accompanies the illness and that may even have been involved in the etiology of the disease. *I got this illness because it was meant. The way I have been living my life, I could not have carried on without something happening.* In this sense of the word, the illness brings the meaning with it, and the patient, as it were, receives both together.

Personally, for most illnesses other than those related to chosen (optional) causes such as smoking, I find this a difficult concept to accept. Patients are constantly being encouraged to look for the intrinsic meaning of their breast cancer or multiple sclerosis, when it is quite likely that these are biological accidents that are not predetermined or preselected by the patient. For centuries we have been blaming the patient for a variety of common diseases (tuberculosis, for example), and the idea that all diseases have an intrinsic meaning for the patient's life may be no more than the modern extension of this idea.

However, there is also a sense in which the word meaning can be used to indicate extrinsic meaning – meaning that can be applied by the patient to the illness, and may thus bring some personal meaning to an illness that may have had a random cause. As Viktor Frankel said,[70] the one thing that nobody can take from us is the ability to choose how we will react to what happens. In that sense, the reaction of a person to a biological event (random or not) can be of great meaning in that person's life and the search for that meaning can be of enormous importance. That search – for the extrinsic or applied meaning of an illness – is something we can and should encourage and support. It is something to do with the affirmation of the person's individuality in the face of illness. It is something to do with the meaning of that individual's life. It is something to do with the essence of the human being's humanity. It is something that we cannot ignore if we are to care for that person.

SUMMARY

Patients respond to bad news in ways characteristic of their own coping strategies.

Their responses can be assessed by three criteria:
- Social acceptability (set the limits generously)
- Adaptability: is this helping the patient to cope?
- Fixability: if this is not helping, can you intervene to help, and if not, can someone else?

In the event of conflict, try to
- Step back and not be swayed by the conflict itself
- "Act, not react"
- Define areas that cannot be resolved

This chapter lists twenty major categories of patients' reactions, but perhaps the most consistently useful tips are:
- If the patient cries, offer a handkerchief or tissue.
- With children, get help sooner rather than later.

FURTHER READING

Bendix T. The anxious patient – Therapeutic dialogue in practice. London: Livingstone, 1982

6 Other Peoples' Reactions

Reactions of family and friends

FAMILY AND FRIENDS: SOME GENERAL COMMENTS

In most clinical situations the family members and the friends of the patient are part (often an important one) of the setting in which the patient responds to bad news and faces the illness. Emotions of considerable strength and force are frequently expressed by family members, and this is perhaps not surprising. In some respects, the bonds between people are most clearly revealed when they are threatened, and the strength of the emotion displayed by a family member is almost always a sign of the strength of the bond between her or him and the patient.

It is also worth noting that bonds may be very strong even if communication between family members is poor or totally absent. A son who does not speak to his father for twenty years is exhibiting a very strong (but not healthy or functional) bond to the father. It takes a major and continued effort to maintain such a silence for a long time, and if the father then falls ill there might well be very strong emotions (including guilt and anger, for example) expressed by the son despite or because of the long estrangement.

As with any aspect of the patient's world, family members can make things better for the patient or they can make them worse. When they are helpful, family members can be the most useful allies the health care team can ever have; when they are unhelpful, they may create greater problems than the patient ever can.

> **Ground Rule: The stronger the family ties (helpful or unhelpful), the more intense will be the family's reactions (helpful or unhelpful).**

Because of the frequency and intensity of reactions by family members, it is important to have some general principles in handling them.

Your primary responsibility

It is of singular importance to remember that, whatever the family members say or do, if the patient is mentally competent your primary responsibility is for the patient's welfare and nobody else's. If there is a conflict between the wishes and the rights of the patient and those of the family (providing the patient is not mentally incompetent and unable to make decisions), your obligation is to uphold the patient's rights and choices first of all. This principle may seem obvious, but in the heat of the moment, particularly when the patient is sick and distressed and the family members are healthy and articulate, it is easy to forget with whose interests the professional's responsibilities lie.

> **Ground Rule: If the patient is mentally competent, your primary obligation is to uphold the rights and choices of the patient, not the family.**

The family as context

Having stated that the patient is the professional's primary responsibility, it must immediately be emphasized that the family members are (usually) a significant part of the context in which the patient faces the threat of illness, and whenever possible you should try to organize the situation so that everyone involved shares the same objectives.

Ground Rule: Even though they have a lower priority than the patient, family members may be very important. Whenever possible try and work with them, not against them.

Rules for sharing bad news with family members

Obtain the patient's consent: If the patient is mentally competent, then there is an ethical (and legal) obligation on any health care professional to obtain the patient's consent before sharing any information about the patient's medical condition with a friend or family member. If there is another person with the patient when you start an interview about bad news, ascertain the person's relationship with the patient (see chapter 4, "Who Should Be There?") and find out if the patient would like the other person to be present during the interview.

There are two ways of doing this. You may either ask the patient with the person present (*Would you like your husband to stay while we talk?*) or, if your prefer, you can ask the family member to leave for a moment and then ask the patient privately if he or she would like the person present. It is usually easier to use the former method unless you detect an atmosphere of antagonism between the patient and family member. If a relative requests a separate interview with you, you must seek the permission of the patient first (and preferably make a written note of that permission). Occasionally you can get caught off guard:

> **Case History:** Sarah H. was a woman of 39 who had chronic aggressive hepatitis and was seriously ill, although not near the end of her life. Her physician received a phone call from Sarah's mother, who wanted to know the prognosis and how long Sarah would live. Something in the mother's voice made the doctor suspicious that the mother was too enthusiastic to know the details. He asked what Sarah had told the mother, who replied that Sarah would not discuss it. The doctor at once went to Sarah's ward, where he found the mother hovering near the bedside: she had been phoning from the ward-phone. Sarah was extremely angry. The mother was actually Sarah's adoptive mother, and Sarah had told her that she was not leaving her anything in her will since they had had a bad relationship

for decades. The mother was trying to persuade Sarah to change her will and was prepared to use the information about the prognosis as emotional leverage. Had the physician given the information he would have been vulnerable to major criticism (and even legal action) from Sarah.

If the patient is not mentally competent, then you are required to discuss the medical condition with the next of kin. "Next of kin" is a phrase that has a legal definition (there is a hierarchy of relationships starting with the spouse), and depending on the urgency of the situation and the need for discussion, you are obliged to try and contact the "highest" member of the kin. You should check with an administrator (or even a lawyer) if you have any doubts.

Follow the same protocol that you use for the patient: The six-step protocol set out in chapter 4 is as useful for family members as it is for patients. Particularly if you are meeting the family for the first time, do not omit any of the steps:
- Get the context right.
- Find out what they already know.
- Find out what they want to know.
- Share the information, starting from their viewpoint (aligning), and step-by-step bring their understanding closer to the medical facts (educating).
- Respond to their reactions.
- Explain the treatment plan and prognosis, summarize, and make a contract.

As you discuss the medical facts of the patient's condition, the family will begin to respond. Just as with the patient herself or himself, family members may respond with mixtures of emotions or behavior, and those reactions may change over time. On occasions family members may support and encourage each other, and amplify each other's reactions (whether helpful or unhelpful). In other circumstances, they may argue among themselves and diminished a concerted view or participation in decision-making or support. When there are differences between family members, it is important to avoid taking sides; instead, explain as objectively as possible the areas of difference.

If there are a large number of relatives, it is a good idea to ask the family to elect two or three representatives with whom you will have detailed conversations and who will take on the responsibility of telling the rest of the family. Some of the family responses will be of the same type as the patient's responses to the illness (whether the patient is present at the interview or not) and some will not. We will therefore consider the family's responses under those two headings.

FAMILY REACTIONS THAT ARE SIMILAR TO PATIENT'S REACTIONS

Family members may experience any or all of the emotions that the patient can, and any of the responses listed in chapter 5 may be expressed. Thus disbelief, shock, denial, displacement behavior, fear or anxiety, and crying are commonly seen. While these reactions may be selected from a similar repertoire as that of the patient, they may be expressed at a different time ("out of synchrony"). Commonly, you will see a family expressing anger while the patient has accepted the situation, or the family may wish to undertake a guest or may express feelings of guilt while the patient is showing denial.

The reactions of family members that are out of synchrony with the patient may or may not cause problems. If they are the cause of a conflict between the patient and family, you should respond to the patient's reactions as the primary problem, and then respond to the family members' reactions as secondary problems using the same techniques and methods discussed in chapter 5.

REACTIONS THAT ARE UNIQUE TO FAMILY MEMBERS

While some of the family's reactions may be similar to the patient's, there are certain reactions that are unique to family members and are quite different to any responses expressed by the patient. The commonest of these are shielding of the patient, specific types of anger, anticipatory grief, and certain types of guilt and fear.

Shielding: "My mother's not to be told"

> **Case History:** The patient was in her early sixties when she developed hematemesis; gastroscopy revealed gastric carcinoma. The day after the endoscopy, her daughter, an intelligent and hard-working single parent in her mid-thirties, stopped the physicians on the ward-round before we reached her mother's room and begged us not to tell her mother the diagnosis. *Don't tell her it's cancer* she said, on the verge of tears, *the shock will kill her.*   (Continued below)

Every human being wants to protect her or his loved ones from illness, but the sad fact is that we usually cannot. Frequently, however, a family member who wants to help a patient to deal with a life-threatening illness (in the face of their own apparent failure to prevent it) will attempt to do what she or he thinks of as "the next best thing": *If I can't protect her from the illness itself, at least I can protect her from finding out about it.*

The desire to shield others from bad news is clearly a common and deeply ingrained part of the bond between people. It may even be an evolved part of our species' behavior that gives a tribe or group its cohesion and interdependence. In any event, it is a frequent occurrence in medical situations and it is important for us all, as professionals, to think about ways in which the situation can be handled.

In reality, you have to try to achieve two objectives simultaneously: (1) honor the *patient's* right to know, even if the family do not wish it, and (2) *identify* and *acknowledge* the feelings and motivations of the *family* members even if their wishes cannot be acceded to. In some cultures (particularly South American, for example) it is expected that if the news is serious it will be given to a relative and not to the patient; and if that is the way the patient would like to have the information handled, then you must comply with that wish. In the majority of Western cultures, however, patients have a right to information if they want it (and as we discussed in chapter 1, approximately 90 percent of patients want to be told the facts).

Both of these objectives can be met: the first by underlining your responsibility to give the patient information if the patient requests it, and the second by using an empathic response to acknowledge the existence of the relative's feelings and the strength of the bond that those feelings indicate. In that way you give permission to the family member to feel the way he or she does, but at the same time you do not enter into a conspiracy of silence against the patient. Those two objectives were met in a relatively straightforward way in the example of the patient's daughter mentioned above. The physician's reply was so clear that we have quoted it in full:

> **Case History continued:** The patient's daughter was in tears, and the physician in charge of the patient responded with an empathic response: "I realize that this must be awful for you, and that you don't want to see your mother's distress get worse; but even though it may be difficult for you, I have to think of your mother first. If she doesn't ask me what the diagnosis is, and she doesn't want to know, then that's fine; but if she wants to know what's going on, then I am her doctor and I must tell her. I know that will cause her distress – and distress to everyone who knows her – but knowing what's going on may be much less distressing than not knowing what's going on and thinking her family know things she doesn't."

We have set out that physician's response at length, because it was a very clear and simple one and it got straight to the issue, while simultaneously offering acknowledgment and support of the daughter's feelings. Here are some of the other options that might spring to mind.

Scenario: As above, with the patient's daughter

Patient says: *You mustn't tell my mother – the shock will kill her.*

You might respond:

CLOSED QUESTION
What makes you think the shock will kill her? (1)

HOSTILE RESPONSE
What gives you the right to say what your mother will or will not be told? (2)

OPEN QUESTION   EMPATHIC RESPONSE
Tell me what you are most wor-   *(as set out above)*
ried about.   (3)   (4)

---

(1)   In itself, this closed question is not wrong; it is merely counter-
        productive. It is quite true that the shock of hearing a diagnosis
        does not kill patients. However, even though that is a medical
        fact, it will not help the daughter because it ignores her feel-
        ings completely, and indicates that she should not be experi-
        encing these feelings (because they do not reflect the facts).

(2)   Again, this response is factually correct (the daughter has no
        rights that override the patient's), but is extremely aggressive
        and will be perceived as inflammatory and escalatory. This re-
        sponse basically tells the daughter that she has nothing to do
        with her mother's case. Among other things, this response will
        exclude the daughter's assistance (as far as the physician is
        concerned) when, later, the mother's condition deteriorates. By
        taking sole command of the case, the physician is also taking
        sole responsibility for the future – a dangerous position and
        usually untenable.

(3)   The open question here is quite safe. Although it may be very
        obvious what the daughter has been thinking about, this open
        question renders the subject of her feelings a legitimate topic
        for conversation.

Anger

Anger expressed by family members is common and may be directed at one or many different targets. In the following example,
the anger of the relative (the husband) was, if anything, made
worse by the fact that the patient accepted her situation:

> **Case History:** Mrs. Turner was a woman of 58 with a sarcoma
> that did not respond to any therapy. Her husband had bilateral
> osteoarthritis affecting both hips and had had to postpone re-
> placement surgery because of his wife's condition. He came to

every visit and would stand guard by the door, glowering as
anyone came in (even more if he had been kept waiting) and
complaining bitterly and angrily about every aspect of his
wife's care and condition.

First reaction: The first reaction of most of the team was to
feel impatient. His wife was our patient, not him, and we were
all doing our best for her. If he was not part of the solution,
then he certainly should not become part of the problem. We
all had many other patients to look after and it was difficult
enough looking after his wife without his added pressure.

Second thoughts: What we did was to use empathic responses
(as calmly as we could) as early as possible in each interview.
They were almost pre-emptive strikes. While Mr. Turner was
clearly angry, we would talk to the patient and then immediately turn to him (*It must be very frustrating for you in this situation. Your wife is very ill, you have your own serious medical
problems, and I can't give you a definite answer about what's
going to happen next*). These responses identified the emotion
and then gave Mr. Turner overt permission to feel the way he
did. He responded initially grudgingly, but later on with sadness and later still with warmth. He had always been very
close to his wife, and had always been the protector and pro-
vider. His role as onlooker was a new and unpleasant one, and
he needed to be told that her condition was not his fault.

It is also important to remember that several different emotions
can be manifested as anger – particularly fear and guilt. A family
member may be frightened about the impending loss, or may have
feelings of guilt (for instance, about not having been a good enough
spouse, child, parent, or whatever) and may express those feelings
as anger. Hence, the number of potential targets for anger is legion.
As with the anger expressed by patients, it may help you to have
some idea of the range of potential targets in order to help you
identify and recognize the family member's reactions. The unfocused or abstract targets for anger (against the disease, loss of
control, biological randomness, and so on) may be the same for
the family member as the patient, but the focused or specific targets may differ, as outlined in the following table.

A CLASSIFICATION OF FAMILY MEMBER'S ANGER

Against the patient
at the carelessness of the patient (real or perceived responsibility for having brought illness on self); at abandonment (if patient is likely to die of illness); at unfinished business (if provision for family through will or insurance has not been completed); "the Jonah effect" (*Why did you have to bring bad luck [illness] into our family group?*)

Against other family members
old rifts (you were always his favorite); causal anger (belief that friends or family contributed to causing disease), whether appropriate (e.g., AIDS, other sexually transmitted diseases, lung cancer in passive smoker, etc.) or inappropriate; against abandonment or distancing (relatives or friends withdrawing from patient or not visiting more frequently)

Against medical and other health professional teams
against failure of medical science to cure patient; against management decisions (should have found it sooner/treated it differently); blaming the messenger for the news; against loss of control, which now resides with doctors/nurses; against communication gaps (not listening/cold/insensitive/uncaring)

Against "outside forces" or randomness
directed at workplace/occupation (appropriate or inappropriate; may be accompanied by desire to obtain compensation)

Against God
against abandonment (*This death is unfair. I deserve better than to lose my loved one now*)

Impending loss and anticipatory grief

If the illness contains a perceived threat of the patient's death, the family members may respond to that impending loss. The responses may include fear and guilt, and, as we have just said, may be manifested indirectly as anger as well as directly. Furthermore, family members may go through a process of grieving before the patient has died: this is commonly called "anticipatory grief" and is a normal response to impending loss. Many relatives feel very guilty about anticipatory grief (*I feel as if I've already buried him and he isn't dead*). You can assist them considerably by listening to them and reassuring them that anticipatory grief is a normal adaptive mechanism to help prepare for a future loss.

An extremely useful device is to mention the value of bereavement counseling (grief therapy) before the death has occurred. This sends a clear message that you expect the death to occur, and have some possible plans for assistance of the relative afterwards (*If, afterwards, you are feeling really low and might benefit from some help, I'd like you to call me. Some people benefit a lot from some grief therapy, and I can help arrange it for you, if you'd like*). The timing of this conversation is crucial – you must be certain that the relative is near the point of accepting the inevitability of the patient's death.

We will not deal with grief therapy or bereavement counseling further in this book, since there are many detailed textbooks on it already.[71]

Guilt
Guilt experienced by family members is also very common. We all spend much of our lives walking around with unfinished family agendas – things that we mean to say to friends and family, things that we mean to do, and so on. An illness commonly highlights the things that family members have not done and makes them feel guilty (*I knew I should have visited her more often* or *I always meant to tell him how much I loved him*).

One of the most important things that you can do for a family member is to point out that feelings of guilt are very common and that strong feelings of any description demonstrate the bond between patient and family. Furthermore, you can encourage the family member to say the things that he or she really wants to. Quite often a family member said *I want to tell mum how much I love her but I don't know the right words*, to which I usually reply *Well, why don't you say precisely that?* Describing an emotion instead of displaying it (as we have already seen) is surprisingly effective.

Fear
Family members may have their own fears about the patient's illness. They may be afraid for their own future. This is particularly

likely if a parent is dying (*It's my turn next*). They may have pragmatic or financial fears about how they will cope during the patient's illness, or they may have fears (appropriate or inappropriate) that they too will eventually suffer from the same disease. It is worth noting that a family member's fear of illness may commonly be manifested as "somatization," the conversion of emotional experiences into bodily symptoms. You will meet this phenomenon quite frequently: the father has just had a myocardial infarct and one of his children now has chest pain, or the patient has been diagnosed as having gastric cancer and the family member now has indigestion. Even though the clinical setting may lead you to be certain that the family member is not suffering from organic disease, resist the temptation to be dismissive. Follow the rules of effective listening and make sure that you allow the family member to express her or his worries and feelings. After you have heard them you can then be reassuring, telling the family member that somatization is a common and expected symptom stemming from closeness to the patient. Frequently the family member is already aware of the similarity between his or her symptoms and the patient's, and may suspect that there is nothing seriously wrong but wonder whether this is the beginning of neurosis or madness. Reassurance that somatization is common and temporary may relieve that hidden anxiety very effectively.

THE FAMILY AS PATIENT

There are certain circumstances in which the family members may become your primary responsibility (even if only temporarily). The most difficult of those situations is the one in which a patient has died unexpectedly and you have to break the bad news to the next of kin.

"Your husband has died"
The clinical situation in which you have to inform someone that her or his relative has died is one of the most stressful communication tasks imaginable. You are most likely to meet this situation early in your clinical career. This event also happened – early in his career – to one of the authors (R.B.).

Case History: "A 91-year-old grandmother went into septic shock while an in-patient on a medical ward. We diagnosed (correctly) acute appendicitis. She had a large and loving extended family who had been visiting her regularly. She was barely coherent in septic shock and her family wished the hospital to do everything possible for her. She underwent surgery but died the following day. The more geographically distant members of her family continued to telephone the ward for information. Three days after she had died, a granddaughter who had not heard about the death phoned. I happened to answer the phone. She asked how her grandmother was. I knew that I had no idea of how to tell her, but I thought I would try and sound calm and 'professional.' What I said was *Oh, didn't you know? She's died.* The granddaughter gasped and put the phone down. I knew that I had made a mess of the communication, and I wished that I had had some idea of what to say."

Informing a family member of a patient's death is difficult in any clinical setting. For the purposes of illustrating a plan for this task, we have selected one of the commonest and yet one of the most difficult of these situations – a death occurring in the Emergency Department. Often the cause of the patient's death is sudden and unexpected (myocardial infarct or an accident), and it may have occurred during an enjoyable family occasion, when the shock to the family is even greater. Furthermore, you may not have had the chance even to meet the family before you have to tell then the bad news.

There are many different ways of approaching this situation, but we shall set out a protocol that seems to work. You will notice that in order to break the bad news to family members, the health care professional uses a "narrative" approach, starting with a description of the events surrounding the patient's death. Still, if asked at any point in the interview, he or she is ready to confirm that the death has occurred.

1. Get the physical context right

It is extremely important to get the setting right. Most emergency departments have at least a separate office, and many have a special interview room. Use them. The walk to the room may be a long one (though often the relatives are already waiting for you there), but to attempt an interview like this is the waiting area or in a corridor is to invite disaster. Make sure that you and the family members (if they wish) are sitting down.

2. Introduce yourself
Give the family your name and say what you do. The family will probably not remember your name, but hearing bad news from a new nameless face is extremely hard. The introduction will also give you a bit of time and space to adjust to the family. Having introduced yourself, find out who the family members are (*Would you mind telling me who you are?*) and check that it is acceptable for you to explain what has been going on with everyone present.

What you say next depends on your own style, but here is one approach:

3a. If the patient was alive when last seen by the family
If the patient was brought in ill but not necessarily in terminal condition (say, with severe chest pain but still conscious), it is always worth trying to establish what the family members thought of the situation at that time (the equivalent of the patient's Step Two: "Find out what the patient knows"). Since the task is to inform the family of the death, do not then ask them what they want to know (in other words, omit the equivalent of Step Three), but move straight on to give a description of what happened (the "narrative"). Try to make this brief and simple – a family in this situation is not likely to be able to recall very much. Of course, the most important moment is telling the family that the patient has died, and this is often easier coming out of a narrative (*His heart stopped beating, and we tried to restart it, but unfortunately there was nothing we could do that worked. I'm sorry to say that Mr. Thompson has died*). The exact words to be used are a matter of debate. In a clinical setting, there are good reasons for saying *he has died* rather than *he is dead* or the more euphemistic *he has passed away*. The phrase "is dead" may sound a little too detached to a family hearing of the death for the first time. Furthermore, "passed away" is sometimes misunderstood.

Practice Point: Euphemisms can be catastrophic. One story, probably apocryphal, concerns a physician in an emergency department who told the mother of a young man killed in a motor-vehicle accident that the doctors' attempts at resuscitation had been unsuccessful. He then asked permission for an autopsy. The mother saw the doctor in the corridor an hour later and asked him whether the autopsy had been successful and whether her son had recovered as a result of it! Particularly with really bad news, one has to be clear about what one is saying.

3b. If the patient was not alive when last seen
If the patient was not alive when last seen (say in an accident or found dead at home), then do not ask the family members what they thought, but move straight on to give a brief narrative description of the situation as you saw it when the patient was brought in, progressing to confirming the news of the death. In other words, omit the equivalent of Steps Two and Three. (*He had had massive bleeding internally and I'm sorry to say that he was dead when he arrived at the hospital. There was nothing that we could do to revive him.*)

4. If the family interrupts you, be prepared to confirm the death when asked
You are walking a tightrope. You want to prepare the family for the bad news if possible; on the other hand, you do not wish to exacerbate their suffering by spinning out the narrative. Hence you should be ready to stop the narrative if the family interrupts and confirm the death of the patient. In some respects, you need a low threshold for stopping your own description of events and for telling the family that the death has occurred. You may have to return to some aspects of the narrative later on in order to explain why treatment was unsuccessful.

5. Use empathic responses
Empathic responses are your most valuable technique. Use them early and respond to every reaction (*You must be overwhelmed by this*). Be prepared to cope with tears (see chapter 5) or anger or shock. As the family members begin to realize that the death has

occurred, they may wish to be alone or they may wish to see the body (accompanied by yourself, a nurse, or other professional). It is useful to ask them what they would like.

6. Make sure someone is available to help after the interview
If there is only one family member present (such as the spouse, who is now bereaved), make sure that you do not simply walk out of the interview and leave the person alone. Ask the person if there is a friend or other family member in the neighborhood who can perhaps collect the person and look after her or him in the short term. If there is no one, try and find a member of one of the support services (a chaplain or social worker may be available) to stay with the person for a short while.

7. Special circumstances
There are circumstances in which the death is even more tragic for the family (a suicide or the accidental death of a child, for example). In the acute phase, there is not much more you alone can do, but it is important to help the family members take stock of their support systems. It will be perceived as helpful if you ask the family members whether they have a family practitioner, and suggest that they see her or him soon. You can also mention the existence of counseling services and grief therapy.

8. Breaking news of death over the telephone
Occasionally, you may have to inform a family member of the patient's death over the telephone. This is always more awkward than having the interview face to face, but sometimes it simply cannot be avoided if the family lives far away. Granting that the situation is far from comfortable, the following points may be useful:

   a Make sure that you know to whom you are speaking (and don't start breaking the bad news until you know).
   b Introduce yourself carefully and say what you do, indicating whether or not you have met the family member.
   c Speak slowly and give the relative time to adjust (particularly if you are phoning in the middle of the night).
   d Make the point early on that a telephone conversation is

awkward, and that you would prefer to be talking in person. (Acknowledgment of a factor of which you are both aware reduces its negative impact.)

e Fire a warning shot. It is always worth telling the relative that you have some bad news – even using those words (*I'm sorry to say that I have some bad news about your wife*). If the relative interrupts to ask whether the person has died, use a narrative approach to confirm the death. It used to be customary to lie to the family member (*She is seriously ill ... Can you come to the hospital*)? but this invariably leads to distrust and anger when the relative finds out that the patient had died before he or she left for the hospital. It is far better to confirm the truth (*I'm sorry to say that she had died*).

f Ask who is available to help the relative at that moment, and suggest having someone in the house if possible.

g If you are able, offer some further contact. Depending on the circumstances, you may be available when the relative calls to collect the death certificate, or you may be available for a telephone conversation later on. If there is no planned contact, suggest that the person contact his or her own family practitioner later, particularly if he or she is overwhelmed by what has happened.

Separate pathology

On rare occasions, the reactions of a family member are so severe and extreme that you may need to get help for that family member at once. This happens very infrequently, and when it does, it is usually against a background of pre-existing psychiatric problems in that family member's past. If the reaction is extreme, you may have to enlist the help of security services (if it occurs in a hospital) or even call for the emergency services if it happens outside a hospital. In one such instance, a son whom the medical team had been counseling for weeks before his mother's death had a psychotic reaction on viewing his mother's body and attempted to drag the body out of the morgue because he believed that daylight would revive her. This was one of the rare occasions when security forces were required. Such an incident is likely to occur only once or twice in your career, but it is highly unpleasant when it does.

THE PARENTS OF SICK CHILDREN

Parents of sick children carry an extremely heavy load of pain, anxiety, misery, and guilt. Every parent whose child is ill is, to some degree, both the frontline family member and the patient-surrogate. Many medical treatments and interventions cannot be given or performed without consent and are legally the parents' responsibility. Hence, the parents may feel – appropriately – that much of the burden of the illness rests on their shoulders. At the same time, they are affected emotionally by what is happening to their child, and commonly feel (usually inappropriate) guilt because of the implicit "duty" of parents to keep their children free of disease – as if, in some way, a child's suffering is a failure of parenting.

An interview with a parent is therefore simultaneously an interview with a patient (the parent being the legal representative) and family member. It is almost always emotionally demanding, and requires great care and thought in carrying it out. Thus, all the general principles that we have set out previously can and should be applied to these interviews. (In fact, much of the important objective data that we have on doctor-patient interviews comes from interviews with parents, and has been extrapolated to apply to all patients.[72]) To all of the above, then, the following points should be added.

1. Awareness of emotional burden
Be aware that the parent is under exceptional additional strain – including sympathetic pain, anxiety, guilt, frustration, and therapeutic impotence.

2. Stick to the Six-Step Protocol
This is the one clinical setting in which we know of the success of an interview that progresses from what the patient knows or suspects on to the diagnostic news.[73] Do not attempt to introduce information until you have clearly established what the parent already knows or perceives.

3. Need for clarity
In all situations of high anxiety, there is a great temptation to fudge the issues, to back off, or to over-reassure. These responses

are likely to generate more difficult problems later. As far as possible, try to be very clear about the medical facts and about the prognosis, specifying particularly what you do know now, what you will know in the future, and what you cannot know. As you explain the facts of the situation, be aware that you are speaking not only to the supporting relative of a patient, but also to the patient-surrogate. Thus, your response should show your awareness of these two sources of pressure.

4. Use the empathic response
The empathic response is valuable in this setting. If you can increase your own sensitivity to what the parent is experiencing and reflect it back to the parent in the form of an empathic response (whether you feel the parent's feelings are appropriate or not), you will diminish the parent's distress.

5. Aftermath – Obtain help for the parent
(a) Bereavement. In the event of serious illness or death, it is quite likely that you will require some extra help to support the parents. Bereaved (or potentially bereaved) parents carry a heavy burden (the incidence of post-bereavement marital separation is very high), and may benefit from professional counseling or group therapy. It's a good idea to investigate local resources.
(b) Genetic defects. Parents require emotional support, precise information, and planning assistance when dealing with genetic defects in a child. Genetic counseling services are now available in many centers and should be used in all appropriate cases.

Reactions of the health care professional

We have to accept the fact that doctors and all health care professionals are human beings. From the viewpoint of patient care this is sometimes a good thing (because we can offer human understanding and emotional support to other humans) and sometimes a bad thing (because we are inconsistent and our efforts sometimes counterproductive). However, our humanity is inescapable, and while the rest of this book has demonstrated ways of using your human abilities to the best advantage, the purpose of this chapter is to help you to compensate for your human weaknesses when you are at your worst.

We have already seen how empathic responses and understanding of the patient's motivations can help you support the patient and can facilitate the communication and the relationship between you. But what if you don't feel that way? What if you are tired or irritable, or dislike this particular patient, or are intimidated by the patient's anger, or overwhelmed by the patient's fears? The rest of this section will help you to compensate for those feelings (which are frequent and normal) so that even when we do not feel like a Mother Theresa we can still help the situation with what the politicians call "damage-limitation."

THE CONCEPT OF COUNTER-TRANSFERENCE

"Counter-transference" is a term used in psychoanalysis to describe emotions evoked in the analyst by the patient that relate to persons or influences in the therapist's past (in contrast to "transference," which describes the patient's emotional response to the doctor). It is a useful concept because it reminds us that health care professionals are not neutral to their patients, and both patients and doctors react to each other's personalities (whether positively or negatively).

Of course, not all reactions to your patients are to be classified as counter-transference. If, for instance, a patient starts hitting you, you may feel attacked whether or not the patient reminds you of your father! Counter-transference only applies to those reactions that occur because of something that has happened to you previously. However, the concept is a reminder that all of us often will react to our patients to some degree because of our own personal set of associations and experiences. In the majority of cases our emotional responses will be slight and will not be a major factor in the management of the patient's situation. Sometimes, however, the counter-transference will be considerable and may potentially influence your medical plan to a great extent. It may not be possible to prevent those emotions from arising, but being aware of that potential allows us to try to compensate for it.

The causes of any of our emotional responses to our patients lie deep in our own past and experience, and it is not within the scope of this book to prompt a probing at such great depth. However, some patients will remind you of a dearly loved grandmother or the brother you had always hoped for, while other patients will bark at you the way your father did or needle you the way your mother did, and so on. The origins of your reactions are part of the basic material of your own personality. Unless you undertake psychoanalysis you may not reach those roots directly, and this may not matter as far as your job as a professional is concerned – provided that you recognize their existence. In your function as a doctor, you do not have to understand every single aspect of your personality (though it would help all of us if we could). It is only important that we recognize our own individuality and try to adjust for it.

Counter-transference covers the entire spectrum of human emotions: the most important feature for our purposes is the strength of your response, not its nature. For example, a strong positive emotion (finding the patient particularly attractive or intelligent, for example) may influence your management just as harmfully as negative emotions (such as dislike or irritation).

Having given these caveats, the rest of this section will deal predominantly with the negative feelings – whether or not they arise from counter-transference. From time to time you will find yourself disliking the patient or feeling angry, afraid, guilty, or frustrated. Sometimes you will be the only person disliking or reacting to the patient; sometimes everybody will be equally irritated.

WITHDRAWAL

The commonest result of disliking a patient or of feeling guilty, angry, frightened, or ineffectual is that you will withdraw from the patient. Withdrawal can be physical or emotional or both. The following episode is a personal example of withdrawal about which the physician (R.B.) was embarrassed and ashamed – and still is.

> **Case History:** "Mr. Cooper was in his early fifties and dying of a pelvic tumor that was fungating through his lower abdominal

wall. The senior staff surgeon had told him that nothing could be done, following which ward-round visits were perfunctory. The residents were always busy and, as the intern, I was supposed to look after Mr. Cooper's day-to-day care. This was long before the concept of palliative care was widely acknowledged, so there was no available local expertise in the field. It seemed to me that there was nothing to do for Mr. Cooper and nothing to say. I became more and more repulsed by the fungating tumor and more and more afraid of going into the room with nothing to contribute, so I would find excuses to avoid visiting. Eventually the patient sent a message via the nurses to say that he would appreciate my visiting him even if I had nothing to offer. I did visit him daily, but was so bound up in revulsion, fear, guilt, and embarrassment that I was of no use at all. Sadly, there is no happy ending to the story. I let Mr. Cooper down, I knew that I was doing it, and I felt terrible about it. I did not know how to handle the situation, and nobody else knew either. Nowadays I would know how to hold a conversation and I would go in. I suppose that part of my motive in wanting to write a book about bad news is to save the Mr. Coopers of the future from being let down in that way."

Withdrawal can be as blatant and physical as in that example, or it can be emotional: the professional is present, but he or she avoids contact with the patient, and may take refuge in a research protocol or some other scientific activity or avoid eye-contact with the patient by reading the chart.

Withdrawal can arise in many different situations. It may involve revulsion or fear of therapeutic impotence, or it may be caused by anger or dislike of the patient's personality. Whatever the cause, if you find yourself withdrawing from a patient, try to think about what it is that is making you do this. If you can find out what particularly is keeping you away from this individual, you may be able to define some aspects of patient care that you can undertake without withdrawing. (On a personal note, with the patient mentioned above with the fungating pelvic tumor, I could at least have gone in and told him that I was ready to listen even though I had nothing specific for the tumor.)

BACKING OFF

Another frequent response when a patient reacts strongly to bad news is "backing off" – changing the news itself to make it less bad and to reduce its impact (a retraction of bad news that has already been given). Backing off is more likely to happen when the doctor or nurse is relatively inexperienced and insecure. The health care professional gives the bad news, the patient reacts strongly, and the professional then reacts by backing off, mollifying the patient by modifying the bad news (*Perhaps it's not that bad really*).

> **Case History:** Mr. Porter was a man in his late twenties who had been treated for Hodgkin's disease. His disease had gone into complete remission, but two years later he developed treatment-related acute myeloid leukemia, a rare but fatal long-term sequela of therapy. The intern on the team, for some reason, was delegated to give Mr. Porter the news. The intern told the patient that the marrow showed leukemic changes. The patient went into a panic state, breaking out into a sweat and walking up and down rapidly. The doctor reacted to his panic by saying (inadvisedly) that it was only one marrow test and that to some extent marrow reports were subjective. This made the situation dramatically worse and he rushed out to find the senior physician (who probably should not have let the junior doctor handle the interview in the first place). Mr. Porter never trusted the intern again.

Backing off is motivated by our instincts to reduce our patients' distress. However, in such situations the first casualty (to borrow a phrase from Hiram Johnson) is truth; your credibility is the second major victim. It is unfortunate, but true, that although patients may be distressed by hearing news of an illness, they will be much more distressed by the illness itself if they have not ben prepared for it (assuming that they want to know what is going on). For instance, in Mr. Porter's case, if the medical team had decided not to tell him about the result of the marrow test, he would have felt totally abandoned as the leukemia progressed and nobody seemed to know why he was feeling lethargic and had recurrent infections and purpura.

Hence the remedy for the problems created by backing off is simple: prevention. Do not give in to the temptation to back off in order to reduce the distress of the moment. Instead, respond to the distress with empathic responses (or open questions) and acknowledge the existence of your patient's distress instead of trying to wipe it out.

ANGER

Everyone feels anger at some time, even health care workers. Individual thresholds for anger vary enormously: some professionals seem almost incapable of strong anger, while others spend most of their time giving off fumes of bad temper. As several physicians have satirically pointed out, patients have some awkward habits that make their physicians and nurses angry with them – they have illnesses and symptoms, they sometimes do not get better when they are expected to, they sometimes may not be grateful for medical attention, and they may even ask awkward questions.

More seriously, our own anger can be a major problem, and each of us has specific limits. Those limits, of course, vary: some days we can tolerate almost anything: on other days we seem to be primed to explode at the tiniest triggering event. What can we do? The answers are not easy, but the following three steps seem most useful.

1. Acknowledgment
The first step is to acknowledge to yourself that you are feeling angry. In itself, this action may give you a handle on your feelings and may decrease your anger somewhat.

2. Describe, don't display
As with any strong emotion, you do much less damage if you describe it rather than displaying it. As discussed in chapter 5, even when feeling quite angry or impatient you would do better to say *I'm sorry that I am feeling so angry about this* or *I'm sorry to seem so impatient.*

3. If you explode, discuss it afterwards
On some occasions, nothing works and you end up displaying your anger. This happens even to the best psychotherapists, and

the important question is: what do you do next? Probably the best thing is to wait until you are sure you are no longer angry yourself, and speak to the patient about why you felt angry. If you can manage it, telephone the patient the next day and apologize for displaying anger, at the same time explaining what it was that made you angry (thus defining the unresolved areas).

GUILT

Guilt is a very individual emotion: some doctors feel guilty about the most trivial things all the time, while others seem to be totally untroubled by it. Sadly, the medico-legal aspects of patient care are more and more likely to increase the general level of guilt felt by the average practitioner when the patient does not recover.

The physician's guilt is the physician's burden – the problem is that it may intrude into the doctor-patient relationship. If you find yourself feeling guilty, one of the most effective remedies is to discuss the matter with a friend or colleague. The problem is that when we feel guilty we have a tendency to stew in our guilt, feeling ashamed of the initiating cause and then of the fact that we are feeling guilty.

> **Ground Rule: If you are feeling guilty, talk to someone (but not the patient).**

THE "BRUSH-OFF"

A "brush-off," in which the physician deliberately evades answering a patient's major questions, will leave the patient isolated and unsupported.

> **Case History:** The following incident occurred in Britain in the early 1970s. The patient was a Mrs. Sadler, a woman in her mid-sixties with recurrent carcinoma of the colon. The tumor filled much of her pelvis and produced a distressing odiferous mucous rectal discharge. The surgeon was the hospital's senior staff member and had decided to do a minor operation in which he would scrape the lining of the tumor cavity in an

effort to reduce the discharge. On the ward-round, flanked by his juniors, he stood at the end of the bed and cheerily greeted the patient by waggling her toe through the bedclothes. He smiled at her broadly and announced his intentions by simply saying *We'll cure you tomorrow*, following which he moved promptly to the next bedside. There was no discussion on that day or on any other day after that. As the disease subsequently progressed, Mrs. Sadler felt more and more isolated and abandoned. She asked about the prognosis constantly, and if any team member tried to bring her closer to medical reality, she recoiled in horror and shock that the senior surgeon's word was being doubted. The contradictions between what she had been promised and reality made her more and more depressed. Until the end of her life she remained virtually inconsolable.

Ground Rule: Rule for the "brush-off" – do not do it.

WE ALL HAVE OUR LIMITS

Throughout most of this book we have been suggesting methods and techniques of staying in command of the interview with the patient and in control of your own feelings and reactions. In this last section, we have touched on what to do when those limits are exceeded by, for instance, anger. Perhaps the single most important guideline is to get someone to listen to you.

> **Case History:** Mrs. Whiteson was a woman in her early sixties whom we had treated for small-cell lung cancer with high-dose chemotherapy and autologous bone-marrow transplant. The treatment had been a major undertaking and she had barely tolerated the five weeks in hospital, which caused her almost unendurable suffering. However, she had recovered, her lung cancer had gone into complete remission, and she had begun to gain weight and resume her life. Six months after the treatment her tumor recurred. The senior resident knew the patient well and thought that he had the expertise to tell her the bad news. He did so, and Mrs. Whiteson wept uncontrollably. Her misery was almost bottomless. The resident stayed with her

and supported her, and after ten or fifteen minutes she recovered somewhat and left the clinic.

The resident said: "I next remember finding myself in our
social worker's office, though I still cannot remember walking
there. I described the interview and its devastating effects to
her and then asked some trivial question or other about Mrs.
Whiteson's social circumstances. 'Of course I'll take care of
that,' said the social worker, looking at me, 'and, by the way,
you did the right thing in telling her about the recurrence.' I
was taken aback, but as I realized what she was saying I said,
'Now I realize why I came to see you.' I suppose I didn't realize until that moment that I also needed someone to give me
permission to feel terrible about what had happened."

Sharing the burden is a healthy activity and will prolong your
active career as a professional. When there are really painful interviews, talk to anyone who will listen afterwards – colleagues,
other team members, friends – almost anyone except (unless you
are overwhelmed) your spouse. Try to keep your home a sanctuary
from the pressure of work, even if you cannot keep the work itself
away.

There are, essentially, only a limited number of ways you can
cope with your own feelings. You can take them home just as
they are (not a recommended step given the high divorce rate and
domestic strife in medical marriages[74]); you can attempt to drown
them in alcohol (also not recommended given the high alcoholism
rate among doctors); or you can try and resolve them, at least
partially. If you do nothing and just leave them alone, you will
probably do quite well for several years and then suffer from
burnout. It is, therefore, a wiser decision to accept your limitations
as a human being and share some of your burdens with your co-
workers (being ready to listen to some of theirs in return). If there
is one guideline for a healthy and relatively well-balanced career
it is this one:

Ground Rule: If you are getting overwhelmed, talk to
someone. Anyone.

Issues between members of the health care team

WHEN A DOCTOR SAYS "SHE'S NOT TO BE TOLD"

One of the commonest questions that comes up during discussions with medical students and nurses about breaking bad news is *What can I do if a senior physician tells me that a patient is not to be told the diagnosis or prognosis, but the patient asks me?* The more junior members of the health care team are quite likely to be targeted by patients because they are less intimidating than the senior members but are still "in the know" are still perceived by the patients to be part of the medical machine. Nowadays this dilemma is becoming less frequent because there is increasing ethical and legal pressure on physicians to make full disclosure. Even so, there are still some older-fashioned physicians who think that they are permitted to maintain a wall of silence around "their" patients. This authoritarian attitude can make the atmosphere very unpleasant for anyone who is seen to contradict this ruling.

This is not truly a matter of rights (the patient has an absolute right to the information, and the physician has no right to forbid you to answer the question) but one of diplomacy. How can you deal with the situation without having a major argument with the senior physician? The answer is relatively straightforward. Nobody can blame the patient for guessing the situation or for wondering about the true prognosis. Therefore, if you allow the patient to frame his or her own suspicions, you can justifiably relay those suspicions back to the physician and tell him or her that the patient already suspects much of the true situation and wants clarification. In that way, you are presenting the "telling" as a fait accompli (the patient already knows) and you have relieved everybody of the task of telling the patient (and therefore running the risk of antagonizing the physician). In terms of answering the patient here is how it might go:

Scenario: Dr. Baker, the senior physician, has "forbidden" anyone
else from discussing the prognosis with the patient. While you are
performing some minor task, the

Patient says: *So I'm going to die, am I?*

You might respond:

CLOSED QUESTION
What did Dr. Baker tell you? (1)

DECEIT
Of course you're not. (2)

HOSTILE RESPONSE
*Why are you asking me? Dr. Baker
is your doctor; ask him.* (3)

OPEN QUESTION
*What have you been think-
ing?* (4)

EMPATHIC RESPONSE
*This must be hard for you –
wondering what's going on
with nobody to ask.* (5)

DIRECT RESPONSE
I'm afraid you are. (6)

(1)   This closed question is only a temporary evasion. You know
that Dr. Baker has forbidden any discussion and that the patient will tell you that. The patient will then probably repeat
the question – and you will become more defensive.

(2)   Deceipt is counterproductive. You cannot stop the patient from
realizing that he or she is getting more ill and deteriorating as
time goes on. To ask this question, the patient must be thinking about the possibility of dying. By shutting the door on a
conversation about it you are removing yourself as a potential
support for the patient.

(3)   This hostile response also removes you as a support for the patient. As well as exhibiting anger you are also ducking out of
the issue by hiding behind Dr. Baker's "ruling."

(4)   In many respects, the open question is the best option here.
Since you are intending to relay the patient's understanding of
the situation back to the rest of the team, the more clearly you
hear it from the patient, the better. I have placed in this situa-

tion many times myself, and have usually found the open
question the most valuable option.

(5)   The empathic response goes one step further than the open
       question, and in this context it might appear to polarize the is-
       sue (between the patient and Dr. Baker's ruling). Although this
       response is not inappropriate, it might be more valuable for the
       future of the patient's relationship with the team to stick to the
       open question.

(6)   The problem with this direct response is that it will come as a
       great shock to the patient. While it may be better than an eva-
       sion or a lie, you may find it very difficult to get back into a
       supportive role with the patient later.

INTRATEAM MANIPULATION

Health care teams are complex organizations, and it is very easy
for patients to play one member off against another or whole teams
off against other teams. This response to bad news is often a
displacement activity. The patient resents her or his situation deeply
(and appropriately), but diverts that resentment onto the medical
team. One way of justifying the resentment is to feel that "nobody
ever tells me anything" or "everybody tells me something different." The patient may then play a (subconsciously) manipulative
game, blaming the team members for inconsistency.

The only solution to this problem is to have one person in charge
of the informative-giving and have that person tell the others what
she or he has told the patient, and then to ensure that the other
team members do not break fresh ground with the patient, but
limit themselves to taking note of any questions and referring them
back to her or him. Unfortunately, we usually realize too late that
this manipulation is going on – after it has already started. Even
so, if the team members are on the alert, the damage can at least
be limited instead of widening as more and more people get sucked
into the game.

> **Scenario:** The patient, Mrs. Thompson, had recently had bilat-
> eral breast carcinoma. The second primary, coming three years

after the first when she believed herself to be doing well, had devastated her. Now she had abdominal swelling and a pelvic mass. The serum markers suggested carcinoma of the ovary, her third primary tumor. Laparotomy confirmed the diagnosis but her postoperative progress was marked by considerable disturbances. She had constant and major disagreements with the nurses and the gynecologic and medical oncologists, frequently taking excerpts of what one person had said and complaining bitterly and angrily to other personnel (*Why did Dr. Axelrod say he had got most of the tumor, and now you say I've got to have chemo anyway* and *Why are they putting me on antibiotics if they say they don't even know whether I've got an infection?*).

First reaction: Most of us felt, as a first reaction, great irritation. Here was a patient who was doing relatively well medically although the prognosis was guarded. Yet ward-rounds were a battle, and a disproportionate amount of time was being spent on Mrs. Thompson. We were all tempted to close ranks, lay down the law, and "come down heavy" on her behavior.

Second thoughts: The argumentative behavior (to which she freely admitted) shown by the patient was, on reflection, not related to her care but to the devastating diagnosis of her third primary carcinoma at a time when she was disease-free from the first two. We did the following things: (1) we agreed among ourselves that the gynecological team would only talk about her postop progress (and that nobody else would), and that the medical oncology team would only talk about future treatment (and that nobody else would); (2) when involved in an apparent interteam dispute, we would refuse to comment (politely but firmly) on any other physician's management (*I understand what you're saying, but if Dr. Bourne didn't make that point clear, you'll have to ask him in detail what he meant and tell him what you don't understand*); (3) wherever possible, we used empathic responses to deal with her anger (*It must be awful lying here, getting better, but not ready to go home yet, and have different teams and different faces drifting in and out of your room*).

Practice Point: In the event of a major interteam or interpersonal fracas, you can decrease the temperature by clarifying territories and minimizing the number of people who actually transmit sensitive information to the patient. Anybody can, of course, listen to the questions.

In these cases (as in all cases, in theory) it is often worth writing down in the hospital chart a brief note of the information that has been given to the patient. Even something as brief as "I have told Mrs. Brown that the chemotherapy has a 30% chance of causing regression of the tumor" may be of great help for other professionals. Written information does become something of a landmark and fixed point, and reduces (slightly) the apparent sloshing backwards and forwards that the patient can otherwise amplify.

Ethical and legal issues

This is not a book about medical ethics (although we hope it is an ethical book). There are many ethical issues having to do with disclosure and medical confidentiality, and in some respects they represent the cutting edge of medical practice as it advances. Current conventional medical practice itself is governed by law and by current custom (which, for the most part, are in step with each other, although not invariably). Ethical issues arise as the scope of medical practice widens and the number of options available to the patient and to the doctor increases. Thus, ethical issues are almost always bound to revolve around controversies and dilemmas in current practice (*We can not do X – but should we?*). Once they have been resolved, such issues become incorporated into current practice or law (or both) and cease to be "issues." For instance, twenty years ago there were debates about whether the patient should be told bad news or not. Now in modern countries there is no debate. The competent patient has a right to information that we recognize in our current professional practice and that is supported in many parts of the world by case-law. This whole book is based on the principle that patients have a moral right to information that concerns them, and that doctors have no ethical rights to withhold such information.

One important point needs emphasizing about some of the ethical issues surrounding breaking bad news. Many controversies have centered on what is thought to be possible. Often as physicians we search for rational reasons for not doing something because we believe that it cannot be done, which has been true of breaking bad news. Because it had been thought that it was not possible to share bad news with patients without doing them irretrievable and serious harm, it was thought that this should not be done, and that withholding information was justified on the ethical grounds of beneficence. Research data proved those fears groundless: when they were asked, most patients wanted full disclosure and most were dissatisfied if they did not get it. As it became clear that information can be shared without causing lethal damage, the ethical grounds for withholding information become shakier.

However, (as Billings points out[75]) the unthinking stance of sharing all information baldly is as harmful as the unthinking stance of withholding all information (and may indeed represent the same basic attitude). Hence, there is a need for a method of sharing bad news that is based on the individual patient and is sensitive to that person's responses. The ethical question is secondary to the question to technique.

There are, of course, individual ethical issues about sharing information, and there always will be. The finer points of such debates will always belong to the ethicists, but we have to pay attention to them since our future practice may be altered by the resolution of those dilemmas.

Cultural issues

It is difficult to know how much to say about issues that separate people of different cultures. Generalizations are worth very little, since most of the catastrophes (and all of their remedies) depend on a knowledge of the minutiae of the other person's culture.

Case History: An 80-year-old Spanish-speaking man was brought into a hospital in pain and in obstructive renal failure. He had had a transurethral resection of the prostate four years

previously, at which time cancer of the prostate had been diagnosed. His family had decided that this information should be
withheld from him and had prevailed on his physician not to
tell him. Now he was in pain from bone metastases, and the
family, intimidated by him, was again asking his physicians
not to discuss his present condition with him because in his
country of origin it was not the custom to tell the patient when
the diagnosis was serious, but to tell the family only. This,
they said, would be what the patient expected.

First reaction: The medical team's first reaction was to comply
with the family's requests since to do otherwise "might cause
trouble."

Second thoughts: A member of the team raised the ethical issues – were the patient's rights being respected? Since the family was refusing to translate any questions about the patient's
wishes, perhaps the patient's right to information was not
being upheld.   (Continued below)

This case (which is not rare given the large immigrant populations
in every major city) has at least two distinct elements – an ethical
issue and a cultural one. If the patient wishes to have information,
then his rights are being violated (an ethical issue); if, however,
his expectations are that he would not be told (a cultural issue),
then he has, as it were, "decided" to abrogate his rights to that
information. The cultural issue determines the existence (or lack)
of an ethical issue.

Case History continued: The team discussed the patient's
rights and wishes for information with the family. It was
agreed that no information should be given if this was what
the patient wished, and therefore that the patient's wishes
should be sought. A neutral party was selected (in this case the
family practitioner, who had the respect of both patient and
family) who assisted in asking the patient (with the hospital
physician present). In this case, it happened that the patient
said that he was content not to know the details of his medical
condition.

For the successful understanding of most cultural issues, nothing less than a detailed knowledge of that culture will suffice (and sadly this book cannot provide that – nor can any book for that matter). For instance, how can you know (until you find out) that while North Americans think it is rude *not* to make eye contact, Sikhs think that it is rude for males to make prolonged eye contact with females (a problem for North American female physicians looking after male Sikh patients, for instance)? or that among Muslims it is considered provocative for a woman to display any part of her legs or the hair on her head (behavior that may be erroneously labeled "non-compliant" by the physician)?

However, there is one practical tip that may help: when things seem to be going wrong with a person of a different cultural background, it may be due to that background, or, alternatively, to that particular person (there are contrary and cantankerous persons in every culture). It is important to ask yourself *Is it possible that this problem is being caused by a cultural misunderstanding?* The only way to answer that question is to ask another person of the same culture what the expectations would be, and then to get help in finding out what this individual feels. For instance, even though a person comes from the country of Concordia, in which it is generally held that people should not be told anything about their blood tests, she or he might or might not be a typical Concordian. If you are a physician looking after that person you need to be aware of the possibility that Concordians do not like to be told the results of their blood tests, and then you may wish to find out whether your patient is a typical Concordian or not.

> **Ground Rule: If problems occur between you and a person of a different cultural background, they might be caused by cultural differences or they might not. You have to find out.**

SUMMARY

If the patient is mentally competent, your primary responsibility is to her or him.

The family's opinions and feelings are important – but not more important than the patients.

Families can have emotional responses that are
- the same as the patient's at the same time,
- the same as the patient's but unsynchronized, or
- totally different from the patient's.

FURTHER READING

Cleese J, Skynner R. Families and how to survive them. London: Methuen, 1983

Conclusion

As we have said at the start of this book, breaking bad news is a somewhat peculiar part of our job: we all have to do it, but we do not know much about it. As authors, what we have tried to do in this book is to set out a logical and consistent approach that you can use to help patients and family members adjust to medical bad news. We cannot claim that the techniques highlighted are the only logical ones, or that they have been tested in their entirety and found to be the best. However, there is nothing else available. Most of us learned our skills by watching our seniors, and, when there were no role models, we used trial and error (with plenty of the latter). We hope that those days of random apprenticeship and serendipity will soon be over, and that regularized formal teaching will introduce some order and logic into this important part of our job.

Finally, we hope that as you have read through this book you have come to see how important this task really is. If you have ever had a relative who is seriously ill or if you ever been seriously ill yourself, you will know how large the figure of the doctor looms as she or he discusses the diagnosis and prognosis. Even if you know the physician concerned, the emotional tension and the fear of illness make every word and every gesture more significant and weighty. It is no wonder that patients and family members expect a lot us as we carry out this part of the job. The task of breaking bad news is a testing ground for the entire range of our professional skills and abilities. If we do it badly, the patients or family members may never forgive us; if we do it well, they will never forget us.

Appendix:
An Interview Using
the Breaking-Bad-News
Protocol

Note: This is the transcript of a role-play between one of us (R.B.) and an actress who plays the role of the patient. The actress has been trained by a psychiatrist (Dr. Peter Maguire) for this and similar roles, and this interview, which was unrehearsed and unscripted, is the one that is used in the last part of the first of the videotapes accompanying the teaching course (see the end of this appendix). Although this is not, therefore, the transcript of a real interview with a patient, it should be pointed out that in five years of teaching, over a dozen groups of medical students have asked how we managed to film a real patient – despite the announcement on video that all roles are simulated!

Scenario: The patient is a 23-year-old woman with newly diagnosed acute myeloid leukemia. She presented with mild tiredness, some purpura, and a persistent sore throat, and has been referred to an oncology unit after a blood count showed thrombocytopenia. The marrow shows myeloid leukemia, and this following interview with her hematologist/oncologist (lasting just over 17 minutes) occurs shortly afterwards. The oncology centre has the facilities for bone-marrow transplants, and it is likely that one of the patient's four siblings is compatible. At the time the interview was recorded, data suggested that the chance of long-term recovery was thought to be approximately 50 percent for young patients who received a transplant.

DOCTOR: Come in, Miss Brown. Sit yourself down. How are you feeling at the moment?

(Step One establishes courtesies, gets the physical setting right, and starts with an open question.)

PATIENT: Quite nervous, really, I suppose. Well, it's a relief sitting here; they just kept on saying you're going to see the specialist and then find out what's happening ... so ...

DR: You are feeling nervous about what particularly?

(Patient is clearly anxious – cause is not yet clear. Therefore, use of open question rather than empathic response. Cause may turn out to be related to medical diagnosis.)

PT: Well, just about being here, about finding out.

DR: What have you made of the illness so far? What thoughts have been going on?

(Step Two: Attempt to establish how much patient knows already.)

PT: Well, it's been really difficult, because ... I mean, everything happened so quickly.

DR: mmm ...

(Facilitation. Tells patient to continue.)

PT: Well, I mean first I just had a sore throat. Then I began to feel that something wasn't quite right; then it wasn't until I really had to persuade the doctor that I thought I was feeling really funny, not right ... then finally he took the blood test ... and in no time I was in here, and once you're in here you start thinking.

(Patient has presumably seen "Cancer Clinic" sign outside hospital.)

DR: What sort of things have you been thinking?

(Still attempting to obtain clear picture of whether patient realizes seriousness of situation or not.)

PT: Well, it's quite obvious really coming in here; you just see what is happening to everybody, and then I just began to think it was quite serious, really, and the way my family was last night, I just felt that we weren't really talking about anything really.

DR: So you have been thinking that something serious was going on.

PT: Well yes, and everybody just kept on saying that I would just have to see you.

DR: Well, if it was something serious, would you like to talk about it, would you like to know what's going on in detail, so I can tell you what's going to happen?

(Step Three: Asking for clear invitation to proceed with informa-tion-giving.)

PT: Yes, I want to know what the results showed.

(Response is unequivocal – patient does wish to know the diag-nosis.)

DR: Well, the results showed that unfortunately something serious *is* going on. It was the bone-marrow sample that was the major prob-lem; do you remember the sample?

(Step Four: Warning shot, aligning with patient by starting on word "serious" ["I began to think it was quite serious"]. Note historical or narrative approach to the diagnosis.)

PT: Oh yeah.

DR: That was the major problem ... Did that hurt you, the bone-marrow sample?

(Patient has winced at the mention of "marrow sample" – had probably been painful. Important to acknowledge.)

PT: Yes.

DR: Well, it was that that told us just what is going wrong, and it's going wrong in the bone marrow. The disease is called acute mye-loid leukemia. That's a bit like a sort of malignancy or a kind of a cancer in the bone marrow, and that's why you've been feeling so ill, and that's why you had the sore throat ...

(Giving information in small chunks. Patient is silent at end of this, then looks very scared. Patient is already reacting to news. Step Five responses now go on simultaneously with information-giving.)

DR: Sorry, that's a bit overwhelming, isn't it.

(An empathic response based on her facial expression.)

PT: Um ... yes ...

DR: Had you heard of leukemia before?

(Attempting to establish patient's agenda of concerns.)

PT: Yes I had heard of it, yes ...

DR: Well, what sort of things had you heard?

PT: Well, I mean everyone knows the word, don't they? Well, there was a little girl at school, and that's what we knew she had. She wasn't very well really. It was the treatment more than anything else. She just completely changed.

DR: In what way?

PT: After she started the treatment ... I don't know, she just changed, she put on a lot of weight.

DR: You mean she got fat around the face with thin arms and legs.

(Steroids used in childhood lymphoblastic leukemia.)

PT: Yes.

DR: Well, that side of things is probably not going to happen because leukemia in childhood is slightly different ... we'd like to recommend to you that we use some quite powerful drugs, but they won't produce that particular effect. It is very strong treatment that we need to use because leukemia is a very vicious illness; it requires strong treatment to put it into remission. But I think we can be very positive about getting you into remission; there is a very high chance indeed that we'll be able to squash the leukemia right down and get you into remission and healthy life. That we can be very positive about.

(Having named diagnosis, now sketching treatment plan.)

PT: I don't understand what you mean: get rid of it.

(Clarifications of information required.)

DR: What we can't do at this time is absolutely guarantee that we can cure it forever for you, but there is a high chance that we can ... a very high chance that we can squash it down flat and put you into remission with a few initial courses of strong drug therapy. That's what I think we can do.

PT: So when you say its serious, then ... its ... I mean ... I'm not going to die ...

(Patient has shown many concerns about the disease and treatment thus far – now mentions fear of dying.)

DR: Well, you're certainly not going to die in the immediate future. Your chance of going into remission is extremely high. Once we've got you into remission we can see how things go and make a more accurate picture of what's going to go on in the future after that; but there is a very good chance that we can cure it completely ... It's a little overwhelming, isn't it?

(The chance of dying in induction is low in this age group, but the

physician is not ruling that possibility out. Patient is now aware
that fear of dying is something she can talk about legitimately.)

PT: It's just that ... when you know what something is, it's better in a
way ... it's just something that just preys on your mind so much.

DR: Has it been preying on your mind a lot?

PT: Yes, I mean when you come in here, into a place like this, and
they start doing these treatments, and nobody quite says anything
to you, you can't really settle into anything. I've not been able to
settle into anything to read or ... everything, television, it all seems
trivial, rubbish, I just wanted to know ... and now I know ...

DR: Had you thought that you were likely to die in the near future,
was that one of the things going through your mind?

PT: Yes, I guess it was really. I suppose I should feel relieved, but ...

DR: So it's been a very very worrying time all-round.

PT: Yeah.

DR: Well tell me, do you have any folks at home? ... Who do you
have at home that you talk to frequently?

(Starting Step Six planning. Identifying other sources of support).

PT: I'm living with my boyfriend. He's been coming in every day, and
just coming into this place it tells you so much, it breathes illness
on you, breathes bad life, people dying ... and sometimes, with the
treatment it seems to be worse.

DR: In what sense ... in your experience of other people having their
treatments, do you think you will be worse?

PT: Yes, when I look at other people, ... you said it had to be really
vicious treatment; tell me exactly what it is.

DR: Yes, I will. The treatment does have serious side effects, there's
no denying that. First for a short time after the treatments you will
feel sick, nauseated, and we will give you medicines to keep that
down.

(Factual response.)

PT: I've seen people on the wards ... then they need more drugs to
stop them feeling sick.

DR: Unfortunately that does happen sometimes, yes. There's no way I
can pretend it doesn't ...

(Avoiding false reassurance.)

DR: ... but we're getting quite good at getting the sickness down to an absolute minimum. We'll be able to get the right recipe to keep your sickness down.

PT: But I've heard some of them talking ...

DR: Yes, go on ...

(Giving overt permission to discuss anxieties.)

PT: They just say they want to give up, that it's not worth going through it, they feel worse, they just want to leave it all alone, they're being treated like experiments, like test tubes, being pumped full of this and pumped full of that. I mean, I don't know why I am so full of so many questions, really.

DR: Let's take them one at a time now, and seriously. The treatment is very vicious. Some people with some different kinds of cancer may actually feel that it isn't worth it, that the chance of actually getting a benefit isn't worth the cost. But in acute myeloid leukemia, I think I could lay hand on heart and say that if I was in your position I would certainly regard the price of feeling sick as worth it. I certainly feel the chance of remission and the good chance of curing the disease forever are high enough to make that risk, the cost of feeling sick, worth it. I really think that's a fair picture. Do you follow what I'm saying ... does that make sort of sense to you?

(Checking reception of information.)

PT: I suppose so.

DR: What I am saying is that the treatment is not easy, it really isn't, and if I were to say ... this is a doddle [= this is very easy], you'll take it in your stride, don't worry, I'd be lying. I wouldn't be telling the truth. You'd hate me for it. It is vicious treatment, but the chance of it doing you a great deal of good and actually controlling the leukemia and curing it is high enough for me to recommend it to you for a straight course. Well, obviously, I don't feel it's fair for you to make decisions straightaway; perhaps we should talk over this point some more ...

PT: Well, I mean the way you put it ... sounds like I really don't have much choice ... it would be a good idea to have it, really.

DR: I would think so, yes, but I'm speaking personally. I'm just saying what I recommend. But I'm just recommending it; we're not police officers or anything.

(Attempting summary of situation.)

DR: We can only say what we think ... I'm just wondering if it might not be a good idea to perhaps talk it over with your boyfriend. Perhaps you might want to bring him in and we could talk it over together. You may feel less alone that way.

    (Plan for follow-through.)

PT: I think it's a good idea, because I feel I have to look after him as well when I'm telling him!

DR: You feel you have to support him because it's such a shock to him.

PT: ... yes.

DR: What about your mom and dad too?

PT: I didn't tell them until the middle of last week that I was in here. It took me that long, I suppose, to come to terms with the fact that I was in here. So I rung them and they came up and I saw them last night. They're staying with my boyfriend, and they're probably all coming in tonight. Do you want to see everybody together or what?

DR: Well, would you like me to? I'd be quite pleased to see all four of you together; it would be perfectly okay as far as I'm concerned. I mean having more people who are able to support you so you can talk to them later on is fine as far as I'm concerned.

    (Step Six plan is now clear.)

PT: Think that it might be a good idea, yes.

DR: Let's do that tonight, then; I'll talk to all four of you tonight, and obviously there are lots of questions going through your mind, and don't hesitate to jot them down as well.

    (Patient is silent.)

DR: Is there anything you wanted to ask immediately?

    (The final – and compulsory part – of Step Six: Is there anything important that we should discuss now?)

PT: There's just this one question going through my mind all the time, ... Why did it happen to me? *(Patient starts crying.)*

DR: Well, the answer is that we definitely don't know.

    (Physician moves closer and hands patient a tissue. Responds with a direct response – patient seemed to be worried about cause of leukemia, perhaps feeling guilt. An open question might have been as good.)

PT: ... *(crying volubly)* I don't understand it ...

DR: It's pure bad luck. It isn't anything you did, anything anybody did, any poisons or anything else. It appears to be just pure rotten luck. But the important thing is that these days there is a great deal that we can do to put you into remission and probably cure you, and I think you have to hang on to that in this really difficult time.

(Empathic response. Shows that patient will not be abandoned.)

PT: I just have to really, yeah ...

DR: OK.

The teaching videos on which the Breaking Bad News course is based are published in Canada and the United States by Telegenic Videos, 20 Holly Street #300, Toronto, Ontario, Canada, M4S 3B1, and in Britain by Linkward Productions, Shepperton Studio Centre, Studios Road, Shepperton, Middlesex TW17 0QD, England.

Notes

1 Maynard D. On clinicians co-implicating recipients' perspective in the delivery of diagnostic news in talk at work: social interactions. In: Drew P, Heritage J, eds. Institutional settings. Cambridge: Cambridge University Press (in press)

2 de Sorbière S. 1672. Advice to a young physician respecting the way in which he is to conduct himself in the practice of medicine, in view of the indifference of the public to the subject, and considering the complaints that are made about physicians. Quoted in: Katz J, The silent world of doctor and patient. New York: Free Press, 1984:10–12

3 Oken D. What to tell cancer patients. JAMA 1961; 175:1120–8

4 Kline NS, Sobin J. The psychological management of cancer patients. JAMA 1951; 146:1547–51

5 Pratt L, Seligman A, Reader RU. Physicians' views on the level of medical information among patients. Am J Public Health 1957; 47:1277–83

6 Hinton J. Whom do dying patients tell? BR Med J 1980; 281:1328–30

7 Finesinger JE, Shands HC, Abrams RP. Managing emotional problems of cancer patient. CA Bull Can Prog 1953; 3:19–31

8 Mackenzie TB, Popkin MK. Suicide in the medical patient. Int J Psychiatry in Medicine 1987; 17:3–22

9 Jones S. Telling the right patient. Brit Med J 1981; 283:291–2. Henriques B, Stadil F, Baden H. Patient information about cancer. Acta Chir Scan 1980d; 146:309–11. Cassileth BR, Zupkis RV, Sutton-Smith K, March V. Information and participation preferences among cancer patients. Ann Int Med 1980; 92:832–6

10 Ley P. Communicating with patients – improving communication satisfaction and compliance. London: Croom Helm, 1988. Kelly WD, Friesen SR. Do cancer patients want to be told? Surgery 1950; 27:822–6

11 McIntosh J. Processes of communication, information seeking and control associated with cancer – a selective review of the literature. Soc Sci Med 1974; 8:167–87

12 Northouse P, Northouse LLO. Communication and cancer: issues confronting patients, health professionals and family members. J Psychosocial Onc 1987; 5:17–45

13 Novack DH, Plumer R, Smith RL, et al. Changes in physicians' attitudes toward telling the cancer patient. JAMA 1979; 241:897–900

14 Billings A. Sharing bad news in out-patient management of advanced malignancy. Philadelphia: Lippincott, 1985

15 Maynard D. Bearing bad news in clinical settings. In: Dervin B, ed. Progress in communication sciences. Norwood: Ablex, 1991

16 Anonymous. In cancer, honesty is here to stay [Editorial]. Lancet 1980; 1:245

17 Simpson MA. Therapeutic uses of truth in the dying patient (Wilkes E, ed.). Lancaster: MTP Press, 1982:255–62

18 Buckman R. Breaking bad news – why is it still so difficult? Br Med J 1984; 288:1597–9

19 Reiser DE, Schroder AK. Patient interviewing: the human dimension. Baltimore: Williams & Wilkins, 1980:3–84

20 Buckman R. I don't know what to say – how to help & support someone who is dying. Toronto: Key Porter, 1988

21 Ibid.

22 Kubler-Ross E. On death and dying. New York: Free Press, 1969

23 Becker E. The denial of death. New York: Free Press, 1973

24 Ben-Sira Z. The function of the professional's affective behavior in client satisfaction. J Health Soc Behav 1976; 17:3–11

25 Baron RJ. An introduction to medical phenomenology: I can't hear you when I'm listening. Ann Int Med 1985; 103:606–11

26 Beckman HB, Frankel RM. The effect of physician behavior on the collection of data. Ann Intern Med 1984; 101:692–6

27 Comstock LM, Hooper EM, Goodwin JM, Goodwin JS. Physician behaviors that correlate with patient satisfaction. J Med Education 1982; 57:105–12

28 Stiles WB, Putnam SM, Wolf MH, James SA. Interaction exchange structure and patient satisfaction with medical interviews. Med. Care 1979; 17:667–9

29 Korsch BM, Gozzi EK, Francis V. Gaps in doctor-patient communication. Pediatrics 1968; 42:855–70

30 Hall JA et al. Communication of affect between patient and physician. J Health & Soc Behav 1981; 22:18–30

31 Stewart MA. Factors affecting patient's compliance with doctor's advice. Can Fam Phys 1982; 28:1519–26

32 Barnlund DC. The mystification of meaning: doctor-patient encounters. J Med Educ 1976; 91:898–902

33 Wilson D. Communication and the family physician. Can Fam Phys 1980; 26:1710–16

34 Snyder D et al. Doctor-patient communication in a private family practice. J Fam Pract 1980; 3:271–6

35 Ley P, Spelman MS. Communicating with the patient. London: Staples Press, 1967

36 Dworkin G. Paternalism. In: Reiser SJ, ed. Ethics in medicine. Cambridge, MA: MIT Press, 1977

37 Weston WW, Brown JB. In: The importance of patients' beliefs. Stewart M, Roter D, eds. Communicating with medical patients. Newbury Park: Sage Publications, 1989:77–85

38 Veatch R. Models for ethical medicine in a revolutionary age. In: Hastings Center Report 2(3). New York: Institute of Ethics and Life Sciences, Hastings-on-Hudson, 1972

39 Bates R. The fine art of understanding patients. 2d ed. Oradell, NJ: Medical Economics, 1968

40 Kason Y. Enhancing the doctor-patient relationship in medical interviewing skills course. Year I curriculum handbook. Toronto: U of T Faculty of Medicine, 1985

41 Mount B: personal communication

42 Hall ET. The silent language. New York: Doubleday, 1959 (repr. 1981, Anchor); chap. 10

43 Older J. Teaching touch at medical school. JAMA 1984; 252:931–3

44 Larsen KM, Smith CK. Assessment of nonverbal communication in the patient-physician interview. J. Fam. Pract. 1981; 12:481–8

45 Bendix T. The anxious patient. London: Livingstone, 1982

46 Maynard D. Bearing bad news in clinical settings. In: Dervin B, ed. Progress in communication sciences. Norwood: Ablex, 1991

47 Korsch B, Negrete VF. Doctor-patient communication. Sci Am 1972; 227:66–9

48 Lind SE, Delvacchio MJ, et al. Telling the diagnosis of cancer. J Clin Oncol 1989; 7:583–9

49 Goldie L. The ethics of telling the patient. J Med Ethics 1982;
    8:128–33
50 Jones S. Telling the right patient. Brit Med J 1981; 283:291–2
51 Maynard D. Notes on the delivery and reception of diagnostic news
    regarding mental disabilities. In: Helm DT, Anderson T, Meehan JA,
    Rawls AW, eds. Directions in the study of social order. New York:
    Irvington, 1989
52 Premi JN. Communicating bad news to patients. Can Fam Physician
    1981; 27:837–41
53 Lovestone S, Fahy T. Psychological factors in breast cancer. Br Med J
    1991; 302:1219–20
54 Buckman R, Doan B. Enhancing the quality of life of the cancer pa-
    tient and the oncologist: referrals to the psychologist – who and
    when? In: Cancer in Ontario. Toronto: Ontario Cancer Treatment &
    Research Foundation, 1991:78–86
55 Cassell E. Hope as the enemy [Lecture]. Toronto, March 1990
56 Ingelfinger F. Arrogance. N Engl J Med 1980:1507–11
57 Marks IM. Fears and phobias. London: Heinemann Medical, 1969
58 Greene SM, O'Mahony PD, Rungasamy P. Levels of measured hope-
    lessness in physically-ill patients. J Psychosom Res 1982; 26:591–3
59 Petty F. Depression and medical/surgical illness: "Who wouldn't be
    depressed?" Primary Care 1987; 14:669–83
60 Maguire PG, Kee EG, Bevington DJ, et al. Psychiatric problems in the
    first year after mastectomy. Br Med J 1978; 1:963–5
61 Snyder S, Strain JJ, Wolf D. Differentiating major depression from ad-
    justment disorder with depressed mood in the medical setting. Gen
    Hosp Psych 1990; 12:159–65
62 American Psychiatric Association. Diagnostic and statistical manual of
    mental disorders. 3d ed., revd. Washington: American Psychiatric As-
    sociation, 1987:222–3
63 Mackenzie TB, Popkin MK. Suicide in the medical patient. Intl J Psy-
    chiatry in Medicine 1987; 17:3–22
64 Hietanen P, Lonnqvist J. Cancer and suicide. Ann Oncol 1991;
    2:19–23
65 Evans DL, McCartney CF, Haggerty JJ, et al. Treatment of depression
    in cancer patients is associated with better life adaptation: a pilot
    study. Psychosom Med 1988; 50:72–6
65a Evans C, McCarthy M. Prognostic uncertainty in terminal cancer: can
    the Karnofsky Index help? Lancet 1985; 1:1204–6
66 From the film "Clockwise" (1985) by Michael Frayn, starring John
    Cleese

67 Buckman R. Communication in palliative care. In: Doyle D, Hanks GW, MacDonald N, eds. Oxford Textbook of Palliative Medicine. Oxford: Oxford University Press, 1992

68 Grollman EA, ed. Explaining death to children. Boston: Beacon Press, 1967

69 Slavin LA, O'Malley JE, Koocher GP, Foster DJ. Communication of the cancer diagnosis to pediatric patients: impact on long-term adjustment. Am J Psychiatry 1982; 139:179–83

70 Frankel V. Man's search for meaning. New York: Washington Square Press, 1985

71 Worden W. Grief counselling and grief therapy. London: Tavistock Publication, 1984

72 Korsch B, Negrete VF. Doctor-patient communication. Sci Am 1972; 227:66–9. Maynard D. On clinicians co-implicating recipients' perspective in the delivery of diagnostic news in talk at work: social interactions. In: Drew P, Heritage J, eds. Institutional settings. Cambridge: Cambridge University Press (in press)

73 Maynard D. On clinicians co-implicating recipients' perspective

74 Gerber LA. Married to their careers. London: Tavistock Publications, 1983

75 Billings A. Sharing bad news in out-patient management of advanced malignancy. Philadelphia: Lippincott, 1985